TOTAL-LIFE
EXERCISE BOOK

TOTAL-LIFE EXERCISE BOOK

The Official Japanese Physical Fitness Guide

by Ken'ichi Yoshida
Translated by
Richard K. Winslow, Jr.

A Giniger Book

COLLIER BOOKS
A Division of Macmillan Publishing Co., Inc.
New York
COLLIER MACMILLAN PUBLISHERS
London

Macmillan Publishing Co., Inc.
866 Third Avenue, New York, N.Y. 10022
Collier Macmillan Canada, Ltd.

Library of Congress Cataloging in Publication Data
Yoshida, Ken'ichi, (date)
    Total-life exercise book.
    Translation of Torimu no jissai.
    "A Giniger book."
    1. Exercise.   2. Physical fitness.   I. Title.
GV481.Y59513   613.7   80-18205
ISBN 0-02-082880-2

10 9 8 7 6 5 4 3 2 1

Total-Life Exercise Book was originally published in Japanese by the Japan Trim Association, Tokyo, under the title Exercise for Trim, in four volumes.
Printed in the United States of America

Contents

Foreword

Industrialization, urbanization, and modernization are increasing in almost all societies in the world. A way of life centered on industry and a modern economy greatly benefits the people, but it also creates a variety of problems including "hypokinetic" diseases —degenerative ailments resulting from underutilization of the human body.

An increase in the occurrence of degenerative diseases threatens our health and existence. At the same time, lack of communication in our modern society causes dehumanization. And thus sound human relationships have reportedly decreased in today's organization-centered societies.

Many nations of the world now recognize the value of sports and vigorous exercise. The Japan Trim Association has promoted trim and fitness for fifteen years. This book, first published in Japan under the title *Exercise for Trim,* is one of the representative publications of our association and includes many unique and useful exercises for daily life and work. This book should prove valuable to underexercised people in your country as well.

Yoshimi Furui
President
Japan Trim Association

理事長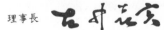

Translator's Introduction

Physical fitness, in both its sources and its rewards, is as much a state of the mind as it is of the body. Evident though this notion may be to the initiated, it is quite foreign to traditional Western civilization. Only in the past ten or fifteen years has the influence of Eastern philosophy and religion had a substantial effect on the life perceptions of many Americans. This influence has come in esoteric forms of religious and philosophic teachings and practices such as those of Yoga and Zen, and in the more physical form of such martial arts as karate and judo.

The present volume is unique in its practical application in modern everyday life of this traditional attitude toward mind and body. The basic problem to which it speaks is both universal and timeless, but it is particularly aggravated in modern industrialized societies: How can one preserve or revive the youthful springs of vitality which reside within the healthy body but which dry up with neglect?

The solution, of course, is exercise, but the programs set forth in this book are special in the spiritual commitment they call for and the close integration of exercise into daily life, into the very corners of consciousness.

The book is directed not so much at the aspiring athlete as at the ordinary citizen, old or young, male or female, student or professional, worker or executive. The exercise programs are not intended to make musclemen or champion runners but rather suggest ways in which modern men and women can retain their health and vitality within the sterile routines of the workaday, impersonal world.

The readers of this book will be aware that it was written originally for a society very different from their own. Japan is a modern industrialized nation which has taken on many ways of the West, yet its social structure remains essentially and fundamentally Japanese. As a result, one will find in this book unfamiliar assumptions about such things as the relationship between an employee and his company, between parents and children, and between men and women.

In particular, the reader should bear in mind that the physical and psychological space allowed the individual in Japan is much smaller than that to which we are accustomed. In part, this accounts for the reputation of the Japanese as selfless, dedicated workers who are willing as a matter of course to give more of themselves to their companies than most Americans could possibly imagine.

Of course, the relationship between the individual

and his company is reciprocal. The company, in return for the devotion and hard work of its employees, is far more paternal in the benefits it provides than are American companies. This explains the presence of recreation leaders in many companies. It also explains the orientation retreat for new employees mentioned in the last chapter of this book.

In this connection, it should be noted that when a young man fresh out of school or college enters a company, he does so with the expectation that he will remain with this same company until retirement. Though of course he is not bound by law, in fact everything in the society encourages him to stick with the company through thick and thin, to become a part of the company family, and to go, if necessary, where his company sends him.

For this reason, a great deal of importance is placed on the transition between school and company and, before that, on matriculation at a college or university which will afford entry to the best possible company. This in turn emplains the severe academic pressure which schoolchildren undergo beginning in the earliest grades.

Japan is a remarkable nation in many ways, not the least of which has been its rapid economic development. The so-called economic miracle of Japan is a complicated phenomenon which cannot be explained simply in terms of this or that national characteristic. But one can observe that there is in Japanese society a strong pressurizing factor, of which academic pressure is only one variety, which speeds everything up and lends a certain intensity to life. One would not want to imply that this pressure is totally without negative effect, but on the whole, it is so carefully controlled by traditional social mechanisms and personality traits that its expenditure is creative and productive rather than explosive and destructive.

I would like to suggest in conclusion that this controlled pressure is directly related to, if not equal to, the kind of spiritual commitment mentioned at the outset of this introduction. I believe that this intangible quality of mind and spirit can be just as instructive to Americans as the many ingenious exercise programs for the body contained in this book.

The Trim Movement

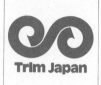

In sailing, the verb "trim" means to distribute the load of a ship so that the vessel sits well in the water, or to adjust the sail according to the wind and the ship's course. By extension, trim can be thought of as describing a human body that is healthy and fit for the long journey through life. In this sense the physical fitness movement originating in Norway in the late 1960s and sweeping through Europe was named *Trimm Aktion* in German. In Japan the English translation became the name of a broad-based fitness movement.

The narrowing scope of physical activity in modern life sets the background for this movement everywhere in the world. Because of today's mechanization, the human body performs less and less, and an alarming drop in physical fitness results. This dark side of modern life shows itself in the so-called civilization illnesses attributable to a lack of exercise. The Trim Movement counters this tendency by shoring up the natural resources of our own bodies so that such illnesses do not have a chance to set in—in the belief

that the best defense lies in the introduction of physical exercise into the ordinary routines of daily life.

The Japanese physical fitness movement began with a government cabinet-level resolution passed in 1964. Since then, the Association for Health and Physical Fitness has collaborated with university researchers and physical fitness experts in developing various studies and programs. At the same time, there has been close cooperation between the Association and various physical fitness organizations at every level of national and local government. Though the Trim Movement was introduced to Japan several years after the government had begun its own programs, the two are now virtually one and the same.

There is nothing more important to happiness than health, and nothing more important to health than physical fitness. Fitness, however, is a private matter which can be effected only by the individual. The ideal of the Trim Movement, therefore, is for the individual to integrate simple but regular exercises into the routines of his daily life. The programs in this book suggest ways that this can be done without the expensive apparatus of a well-equipped gymnasium or the private guidance of a trained counselor. There is nothing difficult or complicated about fitness. It is simply a matter of getting started.

Chapter 1. Testing Your Physical Fitness

PART I. ALL-AROUND FITNESS

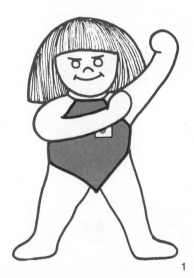

Since the 1964 Tokyo Olympics, October 10 has been designated Sports-Health Day in Japan and observed annually as a national holiday to focus attention on the importance of physical fitness. Each year on this day, sporting events are held all over the country, and physical fitness tests are administered to people of all ages.

Physical fitness, however, means nothing if exercise is limited to one holiday. Nor can we leave its celebration to the heroes of the sports world. Physical fitness should be an everyday affair for each man, woman, and child. October 10 serves to warn us of the threat to health presented by the stresses and strains of modern society. It reminds us of the need for vigilance in the maintenance of fitness. The alarm which sounds each year on October 10 must echo throughout each day of the rest of the year.

A decline in physical fitness is accompanied by no obvious symptoms. It gives no warning as, for example, do the symptoms of a disease. But the detection through a physical fitness test of such a decline invariably leaves one shocked and dismayed. This moment of truth cannot be met with worry and helpless fretting. Climbing any mountain, even the greatest, means taking a first step.

Measure your fitness against the various tasks set forth in the following test. Begin with the tasks intended for your age group, and then see if you can do even better. Incorporate the ones you can't do into a regular exercise program.

1

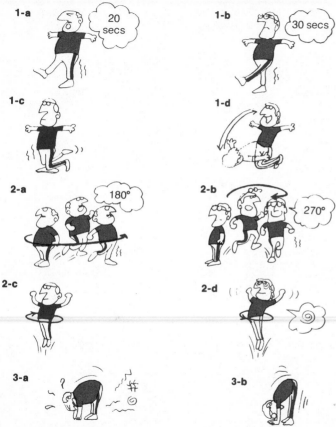

A Simple Physical Fitness Test

The letter "a" following each numbered exercise indicates a task for a man in his fifties or a woman in her forties; "b," for a man in his forties or a woman in her thirties; "c," for a man in his thirties or a woman in her twenties; and "d," for a man in his twenties. Thus, each numbered exercise gets progressively more demanding from "a" to "d."

Balance

1-a. With eyes closed, balance on right leg if right-handed—left leg if left-handed—for 20 seconds.

1-b. With eyes closed, balance on right and left legs alternately for 30 seconds each.

1-c. Kneel for 20 seconds on one knee. Eyes may be open for this, and you may use a towel to protect knee.

1-d. Kneel, bend over slowly until forehead touches floor, and return to original position without losing balance.

2-a. Jump and turn 180° to either left or right, land on one foot and hold balance for 2 seconds.

2-b. Jump and turn 270° to either left or right, land on one foot and hold balance for 1 second.

2-c. Jump high and spin around to either the left or right in a full 360° circle, landing on both feet. Do not twist from waist as you jump, but rather spin with whole body after you have reached peak of jump.

2-d. Jump and spin in a full circle, first to the left and then immediately to the right, landing both times neatly on both feet.

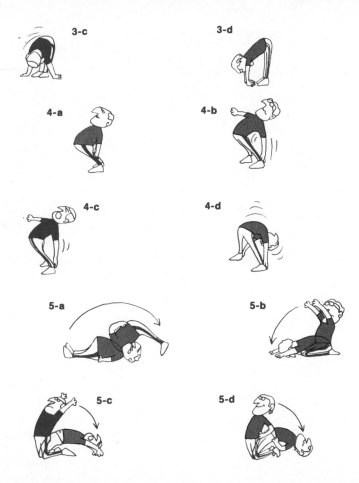

Flexibility

3-a. Keeping knees straight, bend from the waist and touch fingertips to floor.

3-b. Keeping knees straight, touch palms to floor.

3-c. Keeping knees straight, touch wrists to floor.

3-d. Keeping knees straight, touch wrists to floor. Hold the position for a count of 2.

4-a. With legs spread to shoulder width, reach back and touch behind the knees.

4-b. Reach back and touch left heel with left hand, then right heel with right hand. You may bend knees if necessary.

4-c. Reach back and touch left heel with right hand, then right heel with left hand.

4-d. Spread legs wider and touch left heel with left hand and right heel with right hand at the same time.

5-a. Lie flat on your back, raise legs and touch toes to floor behind head, hold for 5 seconds. You may support back with hands.

5-b. In a kneeling position, bend forward at waist and bring chest to thighs as if in Islamic prayer.

5-c. In a kneeling position, bend back and touch floor or come within at least 6 inches of floor with fingers, then return to original position.

5-d. In a kneeling position, bend back and touch head to floor or come within at least 6 inches of floor.

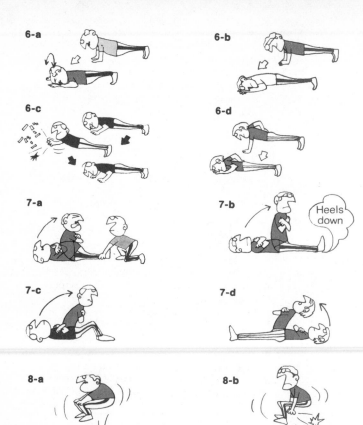

Strength

6-a. In a push-up position with back straight, bend elbows and touch forehead to one hand then the other.

6-b. Cover one hand with the other in a push-up position and touch head to the top hand.

6-c. Do a push-up and clap hands twice. If you can do 3 claps, you are in excellent shape. One clap is not satisfactory.

6-d. Do a one-arm push-up with free hand behind back. Repeat with other arm.

7-a. Lie flat on back with arms across chest. Sit up while someone holds your legs.

7-b. Lie flat on back with arms across chest. Slowly sit up *without* someone holding your legs. Do not let heels rise from floor.

7-c. Sit up with legs bent; do not let heels rise from floor.

7-d. Sit up slowly to a 45° angle without letting heels rise from floor.

Power

8-a. Jump and touch knees.

8-b. Jump and clap hands beneath thighs.

8-c. Jump with legs spread and touch toes.

8-d. Jump with legs together and touch toes.

Heels down

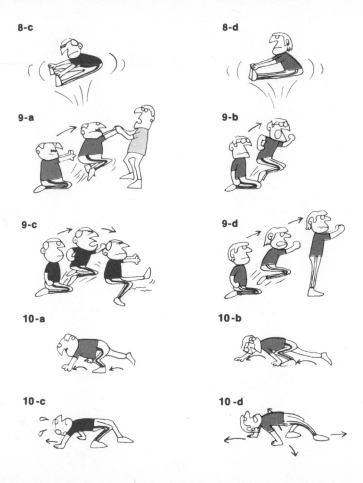

9-a. While someone holds your hands for balance, jump up from a kneeling position.

9-b. Jump up from a kneeling position without help.

9-c. Jump up from a kneeling position, land on one leg and hold balance for 3 seconds. Repeat with the other leg.

9-d. Jump up from a kneeling position and land with both legs straight.

Agility

10-a. Walk on all fours, moving left limbs together and right limbs together.

10-b. Walk on all fours, moving left arm and right leg together and right arm and left leg together.

10-c. Do a crab walk as in drawing, moving left limbs together and right limbs together for 5 paces each. Do not let back sag.

10-d. Do a crab walk as in 10-c, moving 2 paces forward, 2 backward, and 2 to each side.

How did you do? On the average, which exercise age group do you belong to? Is it close to your physical age? Look upon the tasks you were unable to do as challenges to be met in the future. In the illustrations which follow and the accompanying explanations, other tasks are suggested which will provide you with more challenges. Try them.

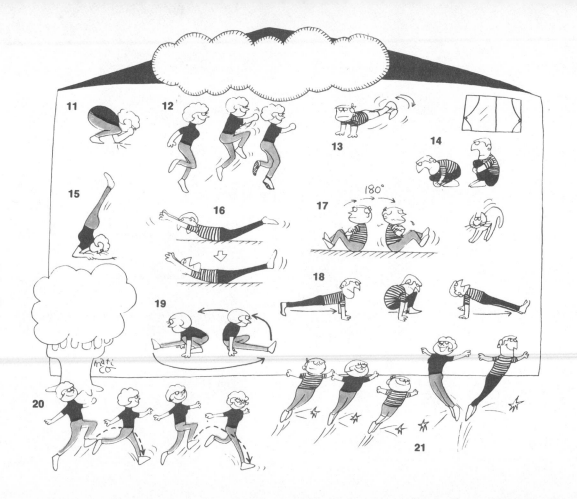

Simple Exercises for All

11. Elbow touching: Spread legs wide (roll pants up to the knee so as not to rip them), crouch, and touch elbows to floor.

12. Jumping crossover: Stand on left leg. Jump and, crossing right leg over left, land on the right leg. Do the same starting on right leg.

13. Double cross: In a push-up position, cross and uncross legs twice while in air.

14. Rump lifter: From a sitting position, clasp knees to chest and pull yourself to your feet. An overweight person will have difficulty.

15. Headstand: Place forehead on pillow and, supporting yourself with arms, slowly raise legs. Do not kick legs up or they will pull you over.

16. Body arch: Lie on stomach with back arched and arms and legs stretched out straight. Turn onto back in a reverse arch.

17. Change of directions: Holding posture shown in the illustration, spin body around 180°. This is harder than it looks.

18. Legs through: From a push-up position, thrust legs through arms as in the drawing. If you have difficulty, try swinging legs forward in a semicircle, lifting one hand to let legs pass under.

19. Foot circles: Crouch on one leg with other leg straight in front of you and turn. A right-handed person will find it easier to move counterclockwise.

20. Hop and spread: Hop off right foot with left knee raised. In midair bring feet together and then spread them to land on left foot. Repeat with right knee raised.

21. Heel clicking: Jump sideways and click heels. Or jump forward and click heels behind you.

If you are able to do all these exercises, you are in quite good shape. But these are meant only to prime the pump. Using a ball, a jump rope, a stick, a towel, or any other object, you can devise innumerable other exercises and games. Devise a program for your family and stick to it.

Chapter 2. Exercise in Daily Life

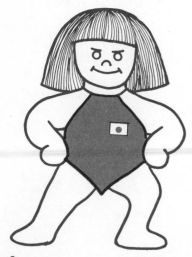

This chapter will show how each person, regardless of sex or age, can get more in physical benefits from the routines of his or her daily life. One way, of course, is to live more vigorously—walking and running faster, jumping higher and farther. Another way is consciously to change familiar habits to make them richer in exercise potential. This might be compared to striking the matchbook against the match.

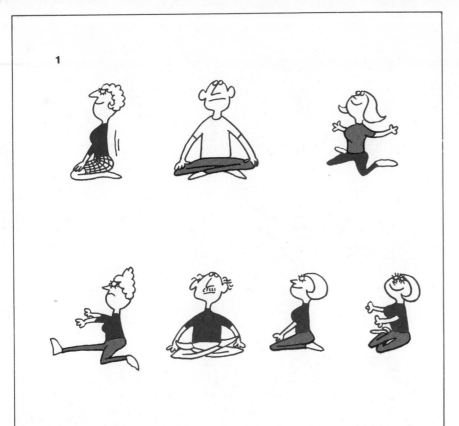

1. Sitting: At home, the Japanese sit on tatami (straw-matted) floors. There is a great variety of sitting postures. On formal occasions, the Japanese kneel, sitting on their heels with their toes slightly crossed. In an informal gathering, they sit with legs crossed. Children often scrunch down with their feet turned out. Some people sit with one leg in front as if jumping a hurdle. Then there is the full-lotus position of Zen meditation, with legs crossed and feet resting soles upward on the thighs. There are also the half-lotus, the side-saddle, and many others. A conscious change in one's normal sitting posture may be difficult, but it also may prove beneficial by stretching and exercising different muscles.

2. Standing up: From a crossed-leg sitting position or a child's scrunched-down position, try standing straight up, raising your arms at your sides for extra lift. From a kneeling position, jump to a stand. Or jump and try to stand on one leg, with the other raised out in front. Another way to stand from a kneeling position is to roll forward onto your hands and then to push yourself back to your feet. Finally, try putting your arms around your knees and pulling yourself into a crouching posture, from which you may then stand.

3. Passing: When passing someone in a narrow place or on a crowded sidewalk, we usually turn our back to the person. If passing on the left (as is most common in Japan), we normally advance the right shoulder and the right leg together. If, however, we turn the right shoulder while putting the *left* leg forward, we give the body a healthy twist. Similarly, there are these same two ways of passing with one's front toward the opposite party. Experiment with them all.

4. Turning corners: On the street, in a corridor, or on a staircase, either walking or running, how do you turn corners? When you make a left turn, undoubtedly your head and torso lean to the left, just as

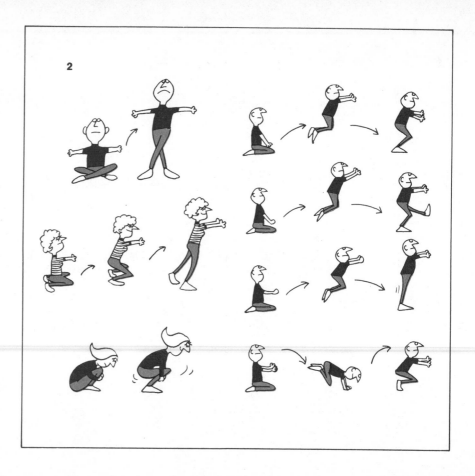

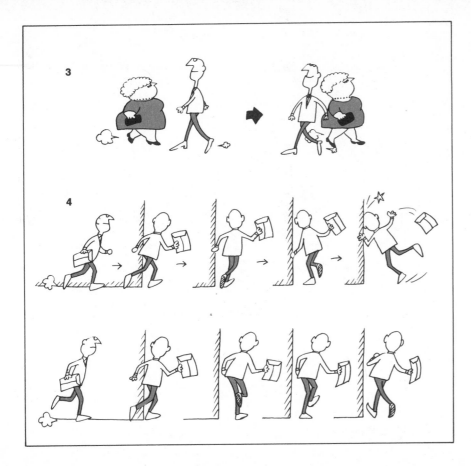

when riding a bicycle. When running around a corner, one counteracts the centrifugal force by leaning the upper half of the body inward, keeping balance by raising the right hand. There is, however, another way of turning which you should consider. This is to lean your head and torso to the outside, forcing the lower half of your body inward and crossing your right leg over the left. Experiment by running or walking in a circle or a figure eight. If you were to slip and fall, the danger of hurting yourself in this posture would be less.

5. Picking something up: Most people stoop at the waist to pick something up. A better way is to keep your back straight and bend at the knees.

6. Passing under something low: People usually stoop forward to pass under the branch of a tree or some other low-hanging object. It is good exercise instead to bend backward.

7. Descending stairs or a hill: Lean slightly forward as you descend. If there are no obstacles in the way, try hopping with your feet together, occasionally coming to a quick stop.

8. Ascending stairs or a hill: Lean forward and take big steps, keeping on your toes as much as possible. Or, conversely, keep your heels down and climb with a posture closer to upright or even leaning slightly backward. When climbing stairs, be sure that each knee straightens as you push up.

9. Riding the public transportation system: When standing in a moving vehicle, passengers usually hold on to a pole or strap for balance. It is easy, when facing sideways, to accommodate to changes in speed, but not to the lateral movements of the vehicle. Conversely, when facing forward, it is easy to adjust to lateral movements, but not to changes in speed. You will find it good exercise to forgo the strap and keep your balance by spreading your legs diagonally, with one foot planted slightly in front and the other slightly behind you.

10. Lifting something: It is sometimes difficult and dangerous to lift a heavy object with just the arms. Bend at the knees and pick it up with your whole body.

11. Putting on socks and shoes: Most people sit to put on socks and shoes and kneel to tie their shoelaces. It will improve your balance and leg strength if you do these things while standing on one leg.

12. Jumping: The running broad jump and the standing broad jump are well known, but there are others as well. Try

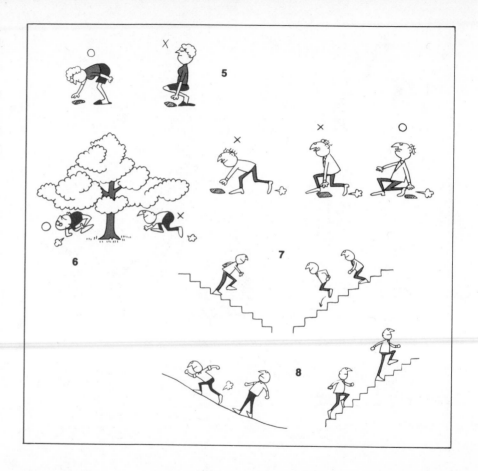

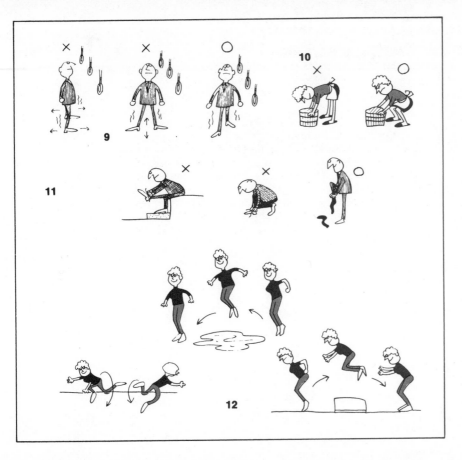

jumping sideways or backward over a low object. You might also learn the roll-over technique for the high jump.

In addition to the above suggestions, you might try walking with your eyes closed (if there is nothing dangerous in front of you, of course!), running backward, and countless other variations on your normal everyday routine. Everything one does can be turned to good exercise. Of course, you should also increase your daily exercise by taking quantitative measures—walking with bigger strides, using the staircase instead of the elevator, and climbing two steps at a time. But it is at the unconscious level of everyday life that the most important changes can be made. And when the time comes to start serious training or exercising, this new attitude toward the details of daily life will be of immeasurable significance. It will also contribute greatly to your will-power and sense of determination.

With this approach to life, think how far ahead you will be if you take up a new sport, and how much quicker you will become adept at it.

Chapter 3. Testing Your Sports Ability

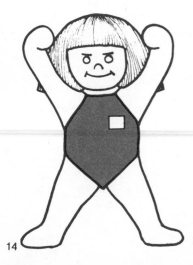

The modern understanding of sports is much broader than it once was. It now encompasses, in addition to the usual competitive sports, such things as actively enjoying the great outdoors; figure skating or calisthenics, which strive for beauty of movement; and walking, running, and other activities which primarily keep one in good condition. In this chapter, you will be introduced to some tests which should serve as an incentive to take up a sport, any sport, at any age.*

*Translator's Note: Because youngsters usually don't think twice about taking up a sport that attracts them, the tests in this chapter are confined to middle-aged women and men who may question their ability for a new sport.

Tests for middle-aged women

1. Interlace fingers behind back by stretching right arm over right shoulder and left arm up from below (or vice versa). If you can't do this at all, you are overweight. If you are in your twenties, you should be able to clasp four fingers; if in your thirties, one finger; if in your forties, you should be able to just touch fingertips.

2. Stand on one leg. Using your hands, raise the other leg to chest. Stand on tiptoe and hold your balance for 20 seconds if in your twenties, 10 seconds if in your thirties, and 5 seconds if over fifty.

3. See how many double jumping-jacks you can do in 10 seconds. Jump and spread legs, at the same time raising arms to shoulder height, then jump to the original arms-down, legs-together position. Jump and spread legs again, this time raising arms overhead and clapping hands, and then jump to original position. In 10 seconds you should be able to do 5 of these double jumping-jacks if you are in your twenties, 4 if in your thirties, and 3 if in your forties.

4. Place three beanbags on the back of each hand and raise arms to shoulder height at sides. Flip hands over and catch beanbags in palms. If you are in your twenties, you should be able to catch all six beanbags 3 times in 3 tries. If in your thirties, you should succeed 2 out of 3 times, and if in your forties, once.

5. Take a deep breath and release it. Then take another deep breath and see how long you can hold it. If you are in your twenties, you should be able to hold your breath over 40 seconds; if in your thirties, over 30 seconds; and if in your forties, over 20 seconds.

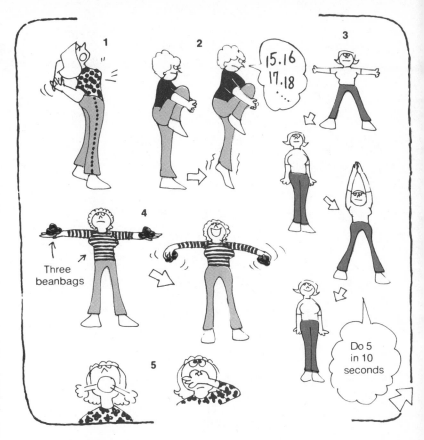

Three beanbags

Do 5 in 10 seconds

15

You should not yet flatter yourself if you have done well on the above five tests. Try the next ten. If you are in your twenties, you should be able to answer yes on seven or more. If you are in your thirties, you should be able to answer yes on at least five, and if in your forties, on at least three.

6. Can you swim 20 m (approximately 66 feet)?

7. Can you do one chin-up?

8. Can you hold a tennis ball in each hand and, with arms raised to shoulder height at the sides, toss the balls overhead and catch them in opposite hands?

9. Can you hand-polish a floor for 10 minutes without stopping?

10. Can you make 5 out of 10 overhand serves (either tennis or volleyball)?

11. Can you jump rope for over 2 minutes?

12. Can you walk for 3 minutes holding a 5-kilo (11-pound) bag or suitcase in one hand?

13. Do you know how to do five different dances (folk or otherwise)?

14. Can you ski or skate?

15. Have you gone on a 25-km (15-mile) cycling trip in the past year?

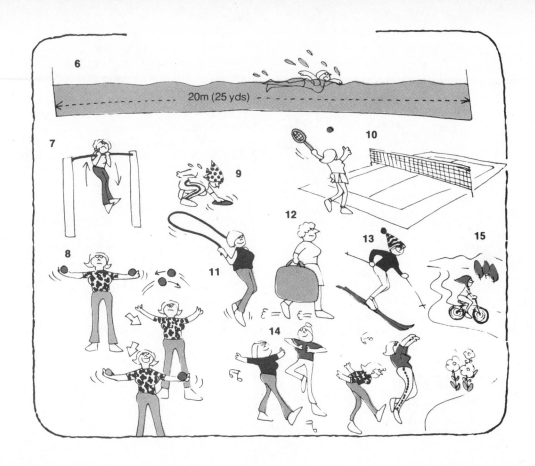

6

20m (25 yds)

7

10

9

8

11

12

13

15

14

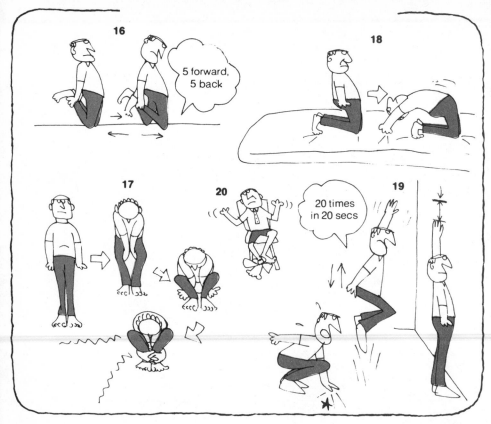

Tests for middle-aged men

16. Holding legs up by the ankles, can you walk erect on your knees 5 paces forward and 5 paces back without losing your balance?

17. Can you interlace fingers in front of ankles as shown in the drawing? (If you are in your forties, interlacing fingers to the first knuckle is sufficient.)

18. Can you bend backward from an erect kneeling position, touch fingers to the floor behind, and return to an erect position?

19. Make a mark on a wall 10 cm (4 inches) higher than your up-stretched arms. Can you jump and touch that mark then crouch to touch your palm flat on the floor 20 times in 20 seconds?

20. Can you sit in a chair and in 1 minute, without using your hands, tie a simple knot in a towel lying at your feet?

If you can't do all of these, you should seriously consider beginning a physical fitness program.

Chapter 4. Improvement at Sports

One can always improve at a sport, no matter how unskilled he or she may be at the outset. Practice brings improvement, and the more you improve, the more enjoyment there is in the sport. Of course, practice takes both time and discipline. It is natural to want an easy way to become good at something, to excel at a sport without undergoing rigorous training. However, practice and more practice is the only way toward improvement, even for the gifted.

In this chapter, I will take a unique approach to the problem. Without denying the need for practice, I would suggest that by sharpening the reflexes and the basic athletic sensibility, the groundwork for improvement in any sport will be laid. It is my theory, as suggested in Chapter 2, that this can begin by consciously altering the simple, unconscious movements of our daily life, often doing the opposite of what we ordinarily do.

A comparison between the novice and the professional shows that the novice expends great effort for little effect, while the pro achieves great effect with a minimum of effort. This, of course, is because the pro knows what he or she wants and the easiest, most efficient way to achieve it.

In our daily lives, we usually walk on level ground, in an atmosphere in which each one of us is the center. We become so accustomed to our self-centered habitual lives that when we are confronted with a different way of doing things, as for example in a new sport, we are quite at a loss. We have to interact with the bodies of other people, with a ball, and with various rules and restrictions. One way to prepare for entrance into such new worlds is to sharpen the awareness of the limitations of our own world and work to expand them. The exercises in this chapter are designed to achieve that end.

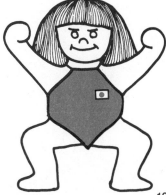

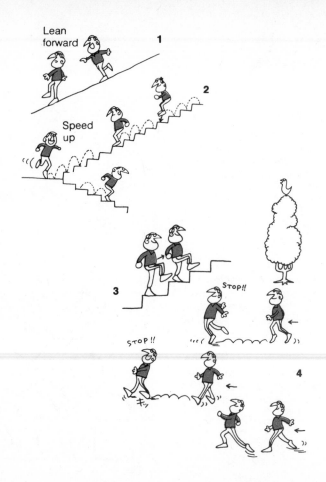

Descending stairs or a hill

1. When descending a hill, lean slightly forward so that you are perpendicular to the slope.

2. When descending stairs, sometimes hop with feet together. When descending in a normal fashion, speed up at the corners.

Ascending stairs

3. Try using only the right foot or only the left foot to advance, bringing the other into line with it at each step.

Ordinary walking

4. Usually, when you are walking and come to a quick stop, you use your toes to stop and keep your balance. Instead, try to keep your balance with your heels when you stop. Also, try turning the instep of the back foot over as you walk. In bare feet or socks, try walking on the outsides or the insides of your feet.

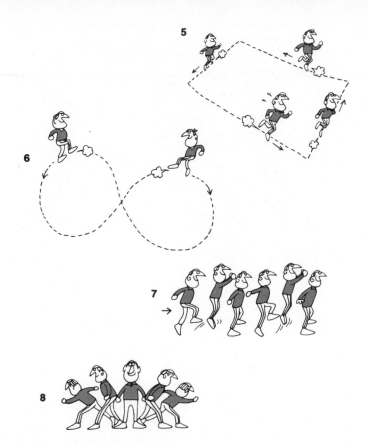

Footwork

5. Imagine a rectangle and run around its perimeter, always facing in the same direction. This will mean running facing forward, sideways, backward, and sideways.

6. Run backward figure eights.

7. There is a children's game which is an effective exercise for adults. Lift one leg, knee bent, and jump with the other. In the air, bring legs together and land with legs spread. Repeat, leading off with the other leg.

8. Stand erect with hands at sides, step forward with right leg, and return to erect stance. Step diagonally to the left with right leg and return to original position. Finally, step all the way to the left with right leg. Repeat in reverse direction using the left leg. Gradually use larger movements. It will be even more effective if you stretch arms at the same time.

Breathing techniques

When you don't have to concentrate on something else, experiment with abdominal breathing as explained in Chapter 22.

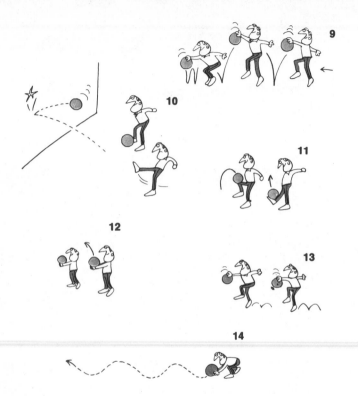

Footwork using volleyball or basketball

9. While running, give the ball 2 large bounces in 2/4 time, then stop and give it 3 smaller bounces in 3/4 time.

10. Kick the ball against a wall, letting it bounce on the floor once before kicking it again. Begin near the wall, kicking with the inside of foot. Gradually move farther away and begin using the toe to kick.

11. Keep ball from hitting ground by dribbling it in the air with instep and knee.

12. Pass, using a volleyball double-handed scoop.

13. Dribble, alternating hands, and skipping once with each bounce.

14. Roll the ball in a wavy line along the floor, never letting it get away from your fingers.

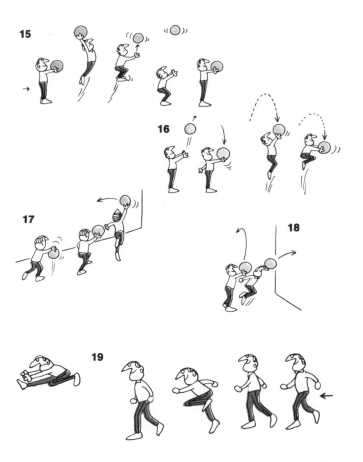

15. Jump with the ball held overhead and, before landing, throw it underhanded into the air. Repeat rhythmically.

16. Toss the ball and catch it with one hand. Also, jump and catch it, both at eye level and at chest level.

17. Dribble the ball along a wall. Jump, swivel, and hook it one-handed against the wall.

18. Using your head, hit the ball against the wall.

19. Another suggestion is to pretend you are a hurdler, and practice the hurdling position whenever you can. Sit in a hurdling position on the floor, or occasionally raise one leg as in the illustration when walking. Practicing like this without the object used in a sport will help you when the time comes to use it.

Whatever you do, get outside and sweat some.

Chapter 5. Simple Isometrics

In Japan, at one time, a man was not considered a man until he could prove himself by lifting a 170-pound sack of rice over his head. How many today can do this? I suspect that there would be many sprained backs if all Japanese were tested with a back dynamometer to see how much each could lift. According to standardized tests, gripping power has also dropped significantly today.

People often ask me how to become strong. Unfortunately, there is a general misconception that strength and even health must be the strength and health of a body-builder. This is not necessarily so. A well-conditioned body may be sleek and supple as that of an antelope. It is true, however, that the all-round training program needs special exercises for developing strength.

Scientifically speaking, there are two ways to build muscles: *isotonic* exercises, which involve the dynamic contraction and shortening of a muscle; and *isometric* exercises, which involve static contraction of a muscle, without shortening. Lifting weights is a form of isotonic exercise. Pushing against an immovable object, such as a brick wall, is an isometric exercise.

Isometric exercises may be performed quickly and easily. Six to 10 seconds of intense effort is enough for any one exercise. In this chapter, I will introduce a variety of isometric exercises which can be smoothly integrated into daily life. One learns them consciously, but they can eventually become unconscious habits.

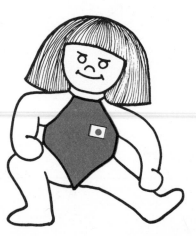

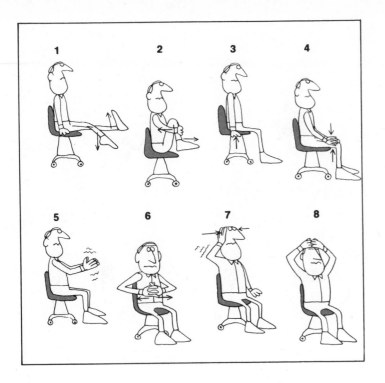

Sitting

1. Sit with legs crossed. Holding the sides of the chair, lift legs slightly, still crossed, and press downward with the upper leg and upward with the lower leg until they begin to quiver. This may be done at work or when riding in a bus or train. Take care not to invite attention by pushing so hard that you get red in the face.

2. Clasp knees to chest with arms and at the same time try to straighten legs.

3. Holding the sides of a chair, try to pick it and yourself up.

4. Sit with hands on thighs. Push downward with hands while at the same time pushing up with thighs.

5. Press palms together in front of you.

6. Lace fingers in front of chest and pull in opposite directions.

7. Push one hand against the side of head, opposing that force by pushing with head.

8. Push forehead back with both hands while resisting with head.

Standing

9. With back to a wall, press arms against the wall. Resist falling forward by straining back and stomach muscles.

10. Push arms forward against a wall, or stand in a doorway and force arms outward.

Strengthening the hand grip

11. Do push-ups on fingers rather than palms. Hang from an iron bar. Squeeze a baseball. When doing laundry, wring sheets by hand. When shopping, dangle the shopping bag from only one or two fingers.

For indigestion

12. Modern man suffers from nervous tension and stomach disorders. Stomach breathing and *shiatsu* massage* are effective against such ailments, because they stimulate the autonomic nerves. For the same reason, exercises involving the stomach are also effective. Two or three times a day (*not* just before or after eating), stand with legs spread and upper torso leaning slightly forward. Pull inward with the stomach muscles so that it feels as if your stomach is up against your back. Maintain for about 6 seconds at a time.

*The reader should consult a book on Japanese pressure-point therapy for further information on this fascinating subject, for example, *Do-It-Yourself Shiatsu* by Wataru Ohashi and Vicki Lindner (New York: Dutton, 1976).

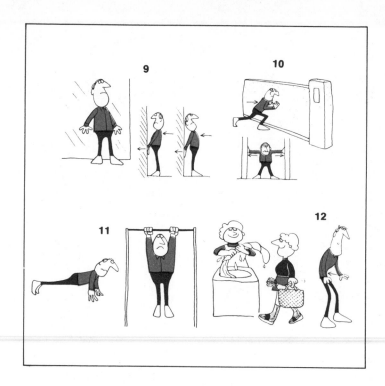

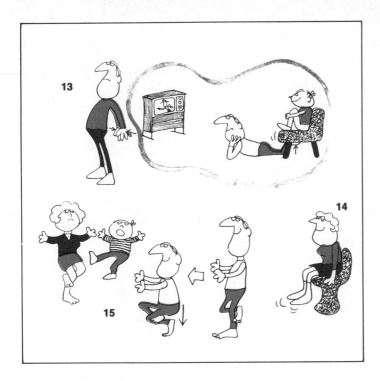

Other ideas

Isometric exercises are infinite in variety and can be done at virtually any moment during the day. For example, try strengthening weak forearms and backs by standing with palms pressed together behind the back **(13).** Or hold one sitting posture for as long as possible without shifting **(14).** Or squat on one leg with the other wrapped behind it at the knee **(15).**

If everyone did simple exercises like these every day, the image of the weak modern man would vanish. If one wants to increase his strength, it is a simple matter of dedication. The time factor is minimal, and once one gets started, the desire to do better grows. More than anything, it is important to maintain a total and balanced program which includes sports and calisthenics as well as habitual exercises worked into the pattern of daily life.

Chapter 6. Endurance

Endurance means not only the stamina required for a 45-minute game of soccer, but also the stamina and willpower to work steadily for an extended period of time—even overnight, if necessary. Tests have shown that stamina, more than strength, flexibility, or the other components of physical fitness, has suffered in modern times. Even in the apparently fit individual there is often a lack of stamina, although this lack may be concealed by agility or quickness.

As our society becomes more mechanized and specialized, the individual grows alienated from his body. His or her musculature in effect becomes obsolete. It is therefore urgent that we take our lives back into our own hands and face up to this potentially disastrous situation.

An important part of the solution lies in the building of physical endurance. This chapter will suggest ways to do that within the context of a daily routine.

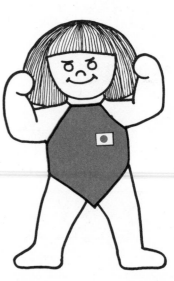

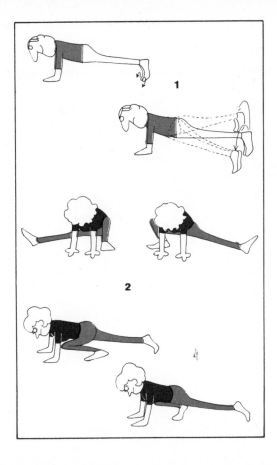

First set aside a 10-minute period each day for some of the following exercises. The benefits will be both immediate and far-reaching.

One-minute stamina drills

1. With hands planted firmly on the floor in a push-up position, hop from side to side with the legs together. Do this rhythmically and make the hops as big as possible. This will improve stamina and strengthen your legs and ankles.

2. For women and others who find the above too difficult, try this: Crouch with hands on the floor and extend one leg, then the other, to the side. For variation, you may stretch your legs in a front-back alternation.

3. Crouch with hands behind your back and see how many times you can walk or hop around the room.

4. If you are shy about running on the street, try running or hopping in large figure eights in your yard. This exercise will also improve agility.

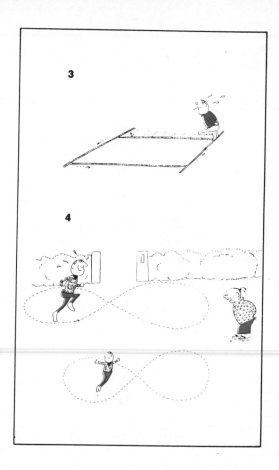

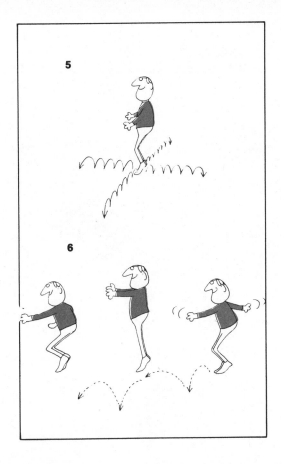

Three-minute stamina drills
5. Hop lightly backward, forward, and sideways.

6. Hop with bigger movements, flexing knees and zigzagging from right to left as if skiing.

Cultivate a more positive attitude toward daily life. Even if you can't set aside a daily exercise period, you will find the following pointers helpful in improving stamina.

7. Shed lazy habits. Instead of depending on others, see to your own needs.

8. Use the staircase instead of elevators or escalators. If you are in your fifties, climb up to 3 flights; if in your forties, 4 flights; if in your thirties, 5 flights; and if in your twenties, 7 flights. Don't use the banister.

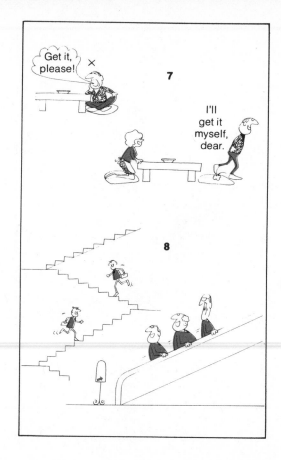

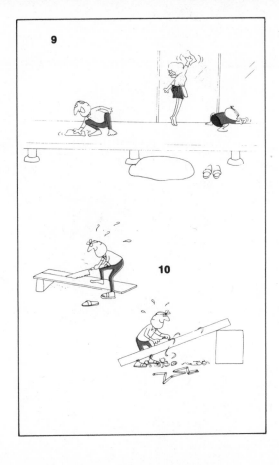

9. Make an effort to help with house chores, and go about each task vigorously.

10. If you are a Sunday carpenter, use hand tools as much as possible, shunning electric-powered gadgets.

11. Before taking a bath, practice the basic movements of your favorite sport until you are sweaty.

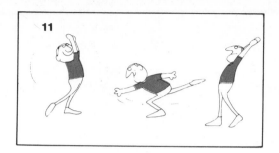

Make time for sports, and afterward be sure to do cooling-down exercises (see Chapter 10). Even if you are exhausted at the end of a game or practice, take plenty of time for cooling-down exercises. These will create a reservoir of energy from which you can draw in a game to display your best form.

Sports in themselves are enjoyable, and if you have become proficient in one, you are not likely to forget the basic skills involved, even with age. However, as one gets older, there is a tendency to compensate for declining endurance by relying excessively on technique. When playing tennis, for example, one tends to give up a point too easily, whereas once he would have run hard to win it. And when a ball goes astray, chase it yourself rather than asking someone else. It is precisely from this point that the road to stamina begins.

Chapter 7. More Fitness Tests

Spring is the season for physical fitness. But before you plunge into some outdoor sport, ask yourself the following questions:

Am I in good shape?
Do I have sufficient energy reserves?
Am I as strong as I used to be?
Have I gotten flabby?
What can I do to get into shape for my sport?

The following tests can give you the answers.

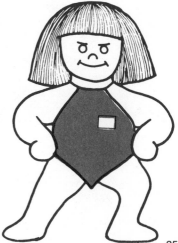

Test 1: Flexibility

Starting position: Hold a broom handle or a pole horizontally in front of you with both hands.

Action: Step over the pole and back with right leg. Repeat with left leg.

Time: 30 seconds.

Points: Each step equals 1 point.

Rest: 2 to 3 minutes.

Test 2: Sit-ups

Starting position: Lie on back with legs straight and hands clasped behind neck.

Action: Sit up so that trunk is at a right angle to legs. Head should touch floor each time you return to starting position. Heels should not leave floor.

Time: 30 seconds.

Points: 3 points for each sit-up.

Rest: 2 to 3 minutes.

Test 3: Trunk lifting

Starting position: Lie facing up with knees flexed and with a pillow in one hand.

Action: Lift trunk with legs, pass pillow underneath, and slide it behind head and around back into the original hand.

Time: 45 seconds.

Points: 1 point for each circuit.

Rest: 2 to 3 minutes.

Test 4: Arm strength

Starting position: Push-up position in front of a chair with a handkerchief on it.

Action: Take handkerchief with one hand and put it on the floor; return it to the chair with the other hand.

Time: 45 seconds.

Points: 1 point for each movement from chair to floor and back to chair.

Rest: 3 minutes.

Test 5: Posture and balance

Starting position: Stand erect with book balanced on head.

Action: Keeping back straight, do deep knee bends without the book falling.

Time: 30 seconds.

Points: 2 points for each successful deep knee bend.

Rest: 3 minutes.

Test 6: Leg and foot agility

Starting position: Stand with handkerchief at feet.

Action: Pick handkerchief up with toes of right foot to thigh level, drop it, and pick it up with left foot.

Time: 1 minute.

Points: 2 points for each time handkerchief reaches thigh level.

Rest: 2 minutes.

Test 7: Stamina

Starting position: Stand in front of a chair, platform, or box 40 to 45 cm (16 to 18 inches) in height.

Action: Step up onto the chair and back down.

Time: 2 minutes (pace yourself; stop if you begin to feel dizzy or ill).

Points: 1 point for each time up and down.

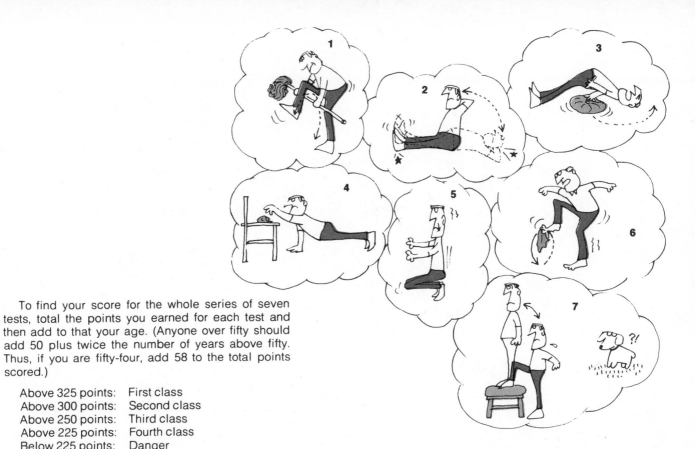

To find your score for the whole series of seven tests, total the points you earned for each test and then add to that your age. (Anyone over fifty should add 50 plus twice the number of years above fifty. Thus, if you are fifty-four, add 58 to the total points scored.)

Above 325 points:	First class
Above 300 points:	Second class
Above 250 points:	Third class
Above 225 points:	Fourth class
Below 225 points:	Danger

A 300-second
program

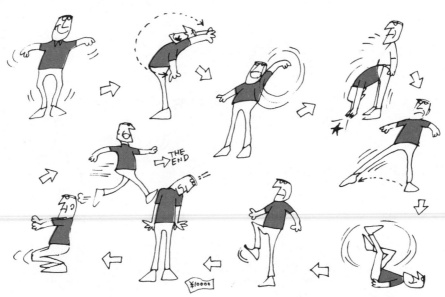

If the results of your test are unsatisfactory, I would like to suggest the "300-second program" described below for use each day to restore physical fitness.

A 300-second program

30 seconds	Relax arms and legs.
30 seconds	Inhale deeply and exhale, at the same time raising and lowering arms.
30 seconds	Rotate arms.
30 seconds	Touch toes, bending at waist with knees straight.
30 seconds	Extend legs one at a time as far as possible.
30 seconds	Bicycle on back.
30 seconds	Lift knees one at a time and turn toes upward.
15 seconds	Touch chin to shoulders.
45 seconds	Deep knee bends.
30 seconds	Run (try to judge time without using a watch).

Chapter 8. Warm-Weather Endurance

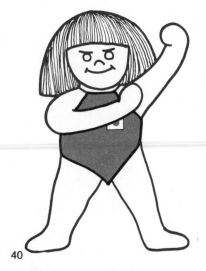

In the heat and humidity of summer, few will heed the call for a vigorous commitment to physical fitness. Lethargy and listlessness set in, and it is all people can do to get through each day. The early morning may be cool, but soon the sun beats down relentlessly, and any physical movement beyond the call of duty becomes tedious. People crave liquid foods regardless of nutrition, and stamina drops off in a vicious cycle of lethargy and poor nourishment.

Mr. Takeda, thirty-eight years old, was the head of the distribution department in a food company which specialized in seasonal products. All year round and especially in the summer, he was so busy that he couldn't even take off two days together in a week, to say nothing of saving up days for a normal summer vacation. To tide himself over the hot weather, Mr. Takeda started a morning fitness program which combined Indian yoga and Chinese *dōin* exercises. And in the evening, on his way home from work, he swam in a neighborhood pool. Many colleagues in his department were so impressed with the results that they began to follow his example.

Dōin is an ancient Chinese form of therapeutic exercise which combines breathing techniques, massage, and passive exercise executed for the most part while sitting on the floor. Yoga, the Indian system of exercises designed to aid in the attainment of Buddhist salvation, emphasizes control of the body, mind, and spirit through breathing and physical exercises combined with meditation.

Without becoming deeply involved in either of these complicated systems, it is possible to benefit from their basic attitudes and techniques. Let us look at the program which Mr. Takeda followed.

Every morning at 6:00 he awoke, sat on the floor in his underwear, and performed the following exercises:

1. With a circular motion, using both hands, rub the area between chest and abdomen 10 times, then rub straight down over the same area 20 times. Next, close eyes and tap teeth together 30 times. Then tap them with finger 20 times.

2. Massage hands, feet, and joints.

3. Make fists and pound the top of head 10 times. Bend forward and pound your back 50 times.

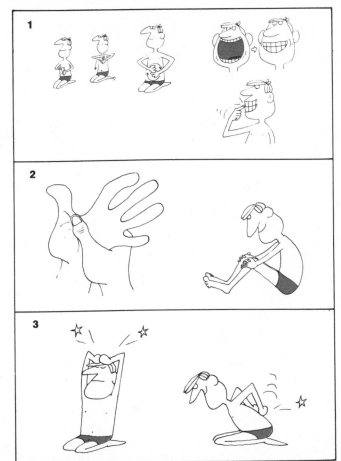

41

4. Lie on your stomach, grasp ankles from behind, and slowly arch back 3 times.

5. Lie face up and slowly lift legs, bringing them over your head and touching them to the floor 2 times.

6. Lying face up, lift legs so that they are at a right angle to torso. Hold that position for 20 seconds by clasping legs just below the buttocks.

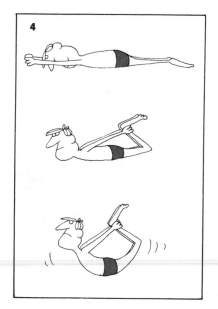

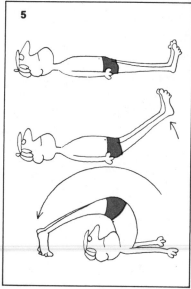

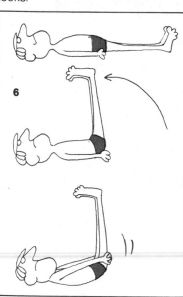

7. Sit upright on the floor with legs straight in front. Bend slowly forward and clasp fingers around feet. (Mr. Takeda was just barely able to touch his two middle fingers together.)

8. Sit in a full-lotus position or simply with legs crossed, and, holding on to feet, curl over backwards and arch back. If you are then able to return to a sitting position, you have strong stomach muscles.

9. Stand with toes pointed outward. Raise heels, inhale, and as you inhale, slowly let body down, knees opening outward. Stop inhaling when buttocks touch heels. Hold breath as you rise back to a standing position, and exhale as heels touch the floor. Take care that upper torso does not lean forward. Do this 3 times.

10. Stand erect with heels together and toes pointed out. Bring palms together (elbows out) in front of chest and inhale, raising palms directly over head. Turn the palms out and, holding breath, bring arms down to shoulder level. Finally, as you exhale, bring arms quietly to rest at sides. Do this 3 times.

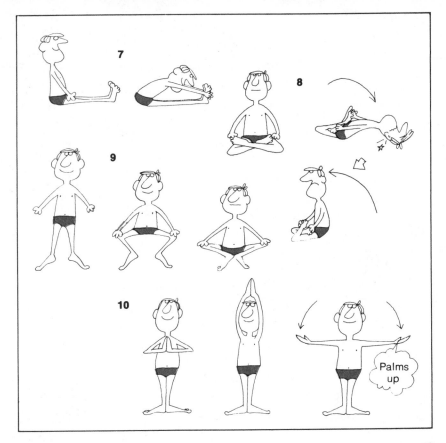

Palms up

Though these ten exercises did not put Mr. Takeda into a state of serene tranquillity, they did put him into good spirits and gave him the appetite for a hearty and wholesome breakfast.

In the evening, Mr. Takeda went swimming. Originally, this was more for relaxation than for exercise, but he was so startled at the drop in stamina since his youth that he decided to work at improving speed and increasing distance.

He began his workout with repetitions of a 12-count warm-up: 1) Raise arms in front at shoulder level; 2) bend them in toward chest; 3) open to left and right at shoulder level; 4) bring down at sides; 5) raise in front at shoulder level; 6) swing back at shoulder level; 7) return to front; 8) bend body forward at waist; 9) do a deep knee bend in that position; 10) thrust legs back into a push-up position; 11) return to a crouching position; and 12) stand erect again.

After warming up, Mr. Takeda swam for about 30 minutes, fulfilling the tasks shown in the swimming workout chart and making an effort to use all the common swimming strokes. The butterfly was particularly difficult and left him exhausted. But oh, how good that bottle of beer tasted at supper.

With Mr. Takeda's positive attitude, the heat of summer can even be welcome.

Swimming Workout Chart
Women

Fitness Level	"Vertical Swimming"	Swimming	Interval Swimming
1	10 times	5 minutes	——
2	15 times	10 minutes	——
3	20 times	15 minutes	——
4	50 times	——	10 25-m (27-yd) laps
5	100 times	——	20 25-m laps

Men

Fitness Level	"Vertical Swimming"	Swimming	Interval Swimming
1	10 times	5 minutes	——
2	15 times	10 minutes	——
3	25 times	15 minutes	——
4	75 times	——	20 25-m laps
5	125 times	——	40 25-m laps

Note: "Vertical Swimming" is a descriptive translation of the Japanese *mogurikko*, which literally means "diver"—not a diver plunging headfirst into the water, but one who is already in the water and goes feetfirst to the bottom of the pool, then springs to the surface again.

During the "Swimming" phase, any stroke may be used.

During "Interval Swimming," any stroke may be used at any speed. If you get tired, you may get out of the water and walk around for a while before continuing.

Chapter 9. Fitness in Winter

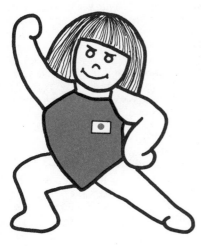

There is a song which Japanese children sing about the dog frolicking in the snow while the cat cuddles indoors by the foot warmer. In cold weather, snowy or not, many people, like the cat in the song, tend to stay indoors. Winter in the city is a season of physical inactivity. Athletic grounds fall into disuse, and everywhere, cold casts a pall over life. Of course, winter sports flourish at skating rinks and ski resorts, but this is more in the countryside and mountains, at a remove from the crowded cities.

Most people consider winter an off-season for physical fitness. The ones who work the rest of the year for one-hundred-percent physical fitness are perhaps the most likely to greet winter as the time for a well-earned rest. But even ten- or twenty-percent effectiveness is enough to maintain health and fitness, as long as there is a basic exercise regimen in each person's life which is as regular and indispensable as washing the face and brushing the teeth in the morning.

Of course, it is only natural that cold weather should be a deterrent even to the devoted. Nonetheless, meeting this test of will is just as important as maintaining fitness. In this chapter, I will introduce exercises and suggest attitudes which are particularly appropriate to the winter months.

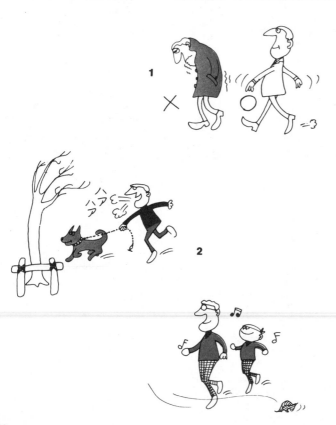

Strengthening resistance

Exercising in cold weather is ideal for strengthening resistance. The old saying that children are open-air creatures is based not only on the fact that children bear up well in cold weather, but also on the medical advice that for their health, they should indeed be subjected to cold weather. Thus, Japanese elementary school boys wear short pants even in winter.

1. Walk erect and tall: Of course, one naturally walks faster in cold weather, but try to cover from 80 to 100 m (add ten percent to get the approximate yardage) per minute. Whatever you do, don't slouch with hands in pocket.

2. Running or jogging: Learn the joy of running or jogging on a winter morning. Running in cold weather is an excellent way to improve stamina. If you stick to a schedule of 20 or 30 minutes of walking and running twice a week, you can be considered a strong-willed person.

3. Jumping rope: Jumping rope is a good alternative to running, but one should not be tempted by fancy rope work such as crossover jumping and double jumping. It is much better to try for speed and endurance as in a boxer's training program. The American Presidential Committee on Physical Fitness has suggested the following five-phase program:

Women

Phase 1	30 second jumping,	1 minute rest	2 times
Phase 2	30 second jumping,	1 minute rest	3 times
Phase 3	45 second jumping,	30 second rest	3 times
Phase 4	1 minute jumping,	30 second rest	3 times
Phase 5	2 minute jumping,	45 second rest	3 times

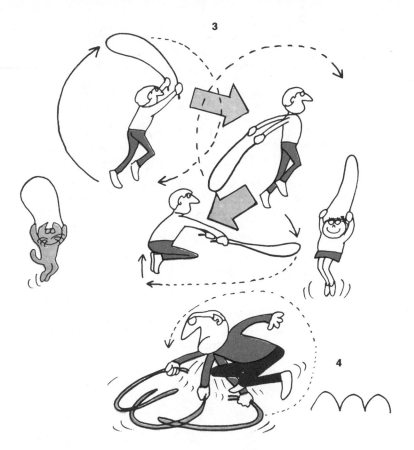

3

4

Men

Phase 1	30 second jumping,	30 second rest	2 times
Phase 2	1 minute jumping,	1 minute rest	3 times
Phase 3	1 minute jumping,	1 minute rest	5 times
Phase 4	90 second jumping,	30 second rest	3 times
Phase 5	2 minute jumping,	30 second rest	3 times

Do not be overambitious. Men, for example, should not assume that they can start with the women's phase 5. Nor should anyone advance from one phase to the next without checking his pulse immediately after finishing a phase to see that it is in the 130-150 range.

There are variations. Try running rope jumping, with a deep knee bend every third step. Also try holding both ends of the rope in one hand and swinging it clockwise (counterclockwise if you are left-handed) under you while you jump over it (**4**).

Staying limber and moving briskly

Cold weather makes the muscles contract, so it is important to do regular stretching exercises.
In the living room or bedroom

5. Squat with hands on floor in front and stretch legs alternately to the sides.

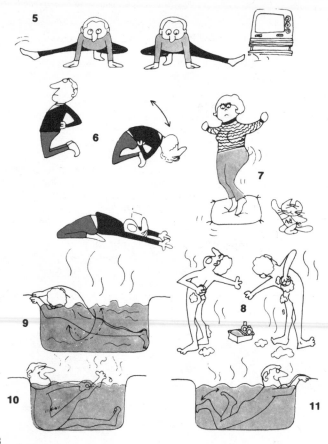

6. Kneel erect with hands at lower back. Slowly arch back and touch head to the floor. If possible, return to the original position, but if not, it is all right to straighten out naturally.

7. Do ski cristies while standing on a pillow. Stand with feet together in the center of a pillow placed on a smooth surface, with toes pointing toward one corner of the pillow. Bend slightly at the knees and turn them alternately to the right or left so that the corner of the pillow moves and straightens out as you flex and straighten knees. At first, you may find it difficult to prevent hips and buttocks from turning as you bend and turn at the knees, but with practice, you can learn to restrict movement to the knees. This exercise will serve as basic training for skiing.

In the bath

8. Stretch well to wash the small of the back.

9. Twist body and stretch limbs while in the bath.

10. Pinch yourself all over to improve circulation.

11. Exercise stomach muscles.

In this day of central heating and other conveniences which help keep us warm, many people lose their natural ability to respond to the environment. Thus it is easy for them to succumb to disease and the various ailments of aging. Of course, as water always flows to lower ground, so humans tend to take the easiest course. But experience has shown the importance for a long and healthy life of active efforts to maintain physical fitness even in the face of cold weather.

Chapter 10. Warming-Up and Cooling-Down

When winter comes, spring can't be far behind, they say. And sure enough, warmer air begins to blow, ice-covered ponds begin to melt, and tiny buds appear on the trees and shrubbery. The human body also wakes up, as if from a long winter nap. This is a time, however, when we must take care to avoid sudden or excessive physical stress. Our bodies need to make the change from inactivity to activity gradually, and gradually back again to rest. In this chapter, I will discuss warming-up and cooling-down exercises.

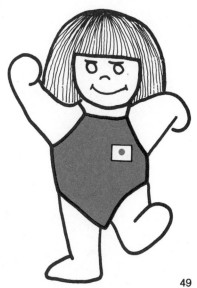

Warming-up

Any kind of strenuous physical activity should be prepared for by less strenuous warm-up exercises. Too often, however, warm-up exercises are limited to deep knee bends, torso stretching, and shoulder and arm limbering. Since these are considered standard, people become locked into the habit of doing them and nothing else.

Tennis players would do well to practice ground strokes and serves in their warm-ups. And when they first get out on the court, they should rally lightly and begin practice serves at 60-percent strength. While for a beginner such basic practice may be an end in itself, more advanced players should consider it a standard part of their warm-ups.

This is not to suggest, however, that the more conventional stretching and bending is meaningless. The following exercises should be included in any warm-up regimen, particularly for middle-aged and older people who are exercising to regain a hold on their youth:

1. To prevent injury to the Achilles tendon: Stand with one leg forward, the other back, and stretch the Achilles tendon by arching back and raising toes of front foot. Repeat with other leg forward. Do this 5 times both right and left.

2. Arm and leg exercise: Do the 12-count exercise shown in the drawing 3 to 5 times.

3. To prevent a pulled leg muscle: Do deep knee bends on one leg, with the other wrapped behind it at the knee. This stretches the calf and thigh muscles and prevents injury. Do the exercise 3 times for each leg.

4. For baseball, first (a) jump, catch, and throw; then (b) slow underhand throws; and then (c) slow overhand throws.

5. For volleyball, first (a) walk 10 steps, turning the back foot over onto the instep; then (b) place left foot forward and slightly to the left with the back foot turning onto the instep. Roll over on the left shoulder and return to a standing position. Repeat on the right side. Finally, (c) jump forward, land on hands, and arch back. Land in a rabbit position or in a push-up position. In this way you can incorporate the basic motions of your sport into the warm-ups.

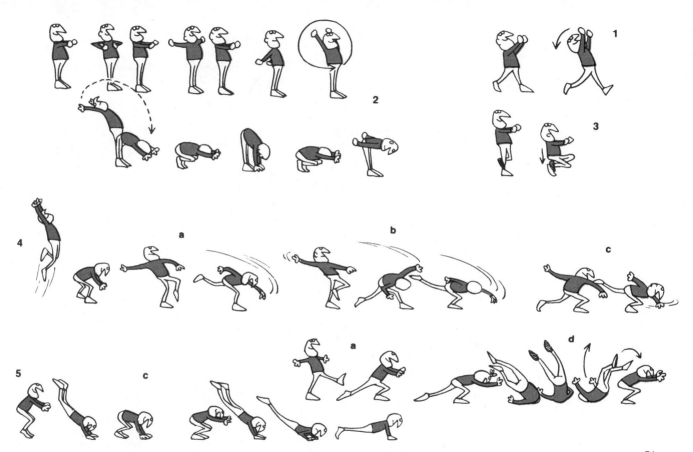

51

Cooling-down

While most people do some kind of warm-up exercises, cooling-down exercises are more often neglected. As soon as the game is over, everyone says goodbye and leaves. This is especially common among older people who exercise only rarely.

When one is engaged in a strenuous sport, the heart has to work extra hard to pump the necessary amount of blood. When the activity is suddenly stopped, the heart continues at this high level, putting undue stress on the suprarenal gland in the kidneys. Cooling-down exercises function to return the heart to its normal state. It is my opinion that the relatively short life span of Japanese athletes is partly a result of the lack of regular cooling-down exercises.

The older one gets, the more time one should give to cooling-down exercises. Ideally, these should be done in decreasing order, from the most demanding exercise to the least demanding. The following is one possible series:

6. Mixed jumping and running: Of course, it is all right to run in a straight line, but figure eights are good because they make you use smaller movements.

7. Torso twisting: Twist several times from right to left. Use your arms to aid the twist.

8. Head or hand stands: If you can't keep your balance, lift legs only partway up.

9. Massage exercises for partners: Stiffness always comes the day *after* exercising. To prevent this, do massage exercises with a partner.

a) One partner lies on stomach while the other vibrates his legs one at a time, grasping the arch and instep of the foot. The vibrations will be felt right up to the neck. It is always a surprise how heavy the human leg is. The person being massaged should keep his legs limp.

b) Normally, when exercising, the body is bent forward, so it is important to counteract this by arching the back. The person lying down extends his arms forward. The partner then straddles his trunk and slowly lifts him by the wrists to maximum possible height, holds him there for 3 to 5 seconds, and then gently lets him down. This is done 3 times.

c) One partner sits relaxed on the floor while the other massages his neck, shoulders, and back.

Reverse positions and repeat the above massage exercises.

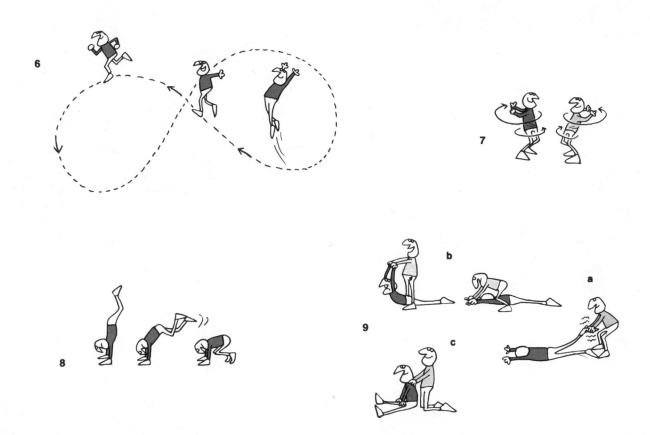

6

7

8

9

b

a

c

53

Chapter 11. Good Posture

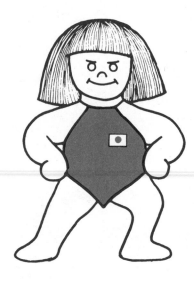

Good posture is not simply a matter of style. It also is a matter of deeply ingrained habit. Miyamoto Musashi, the famous seventeenth-century swordsman, wrote: "The back and neck should be straight, with the chin in, but not stiff. The shoulders should be relaxed, and there should be lightness in the bearing. The eyes need not be piercing, but the heart should see through everything." Musashi's prescription is for the standing body in repose, but it is also the posture from which the body in action may most readily emerge. His ideal is as valid today as it was in the seventeenth century.

Good posture is indeed a matter of habit, but, disregarding the problem of unnaturally bad posture, factors such as fatigue, poor nutrition, listlessness, and long hours of desk work can undermine the foundations of good habit, resulting in poor circulation, headaches, back pain, leaden legs, and a steadily worsening state of health. In this sense, posture should receive more attention then it usually gets in physical fitness programs. The present chapter will attempt to correct this oversight.

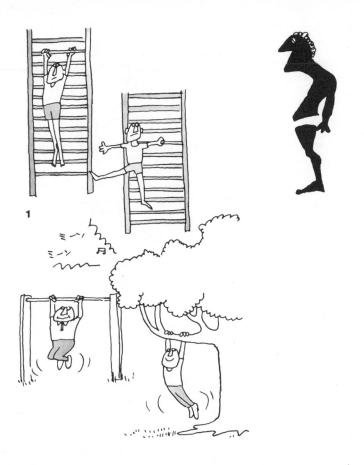

1

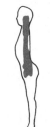

The bad back

Bad posture is typically represented by the so-called swayback, with stooped shoulders, forward-tilted head, an S-shaped spinal column, and a protruding abdomen. It used to be that all gymnasiums were equipped with wall bars from which one could hang and lift the legs, thus strengthening the abdomen. Another remedy, or at least a preventative, for swayback is the Danish-type calisthenic drill.

1. Hanging by the arms: Hanging from an iron bar or a tree limb and doing chin-ups is an excellent corrective to a bad back and at the same time increases both arm strength and stamina.

Types of posture

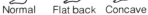

| Normal | Flat back | Concave | Rounded | S-shaped |

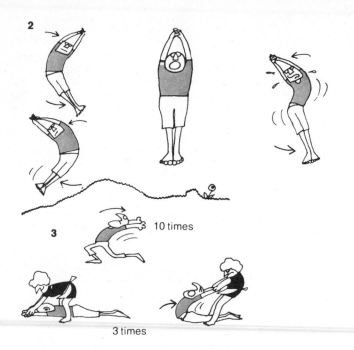

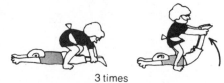

10 times

3 times

3 times

2. Lateral body-bending: Lie on your back with arms stretched overhead, hands joined, and legs together. Swing your whole body from hands to feet, in large half-moons or in an S-shape, first to the right, then to the left. Think of your lower body as the pendulum of a clock, swinging slowly back and forth, and move your upper body either together with it or in the opposite direction. Gradually increase the size of the arcs.

3. Back bends: If your normal posture is stooped slightly forward, you will feel resistance to these exercises, but they will help your posture greatly. Thrust one leg at a time forward and swing your arms and upper torso back 10 times. Also lie face down and have someone pull you up and back by your wrists. Or, conversely, have someone pull you back by the ankles 3 times.

4

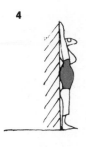

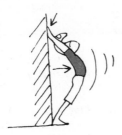

4. Backward wall press: Stand with back and heels flush against a wall and arms stretched up. Arch your back by applying pressure against the wall with hands and pushing out with stomach.

5. Front bends: Place hands on desk with feet spread to shoulder width and back bent forward at a right angle. Without bending elbows, slowly move hips as far as you can to left and right.

5

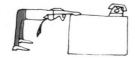

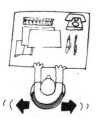

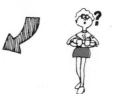

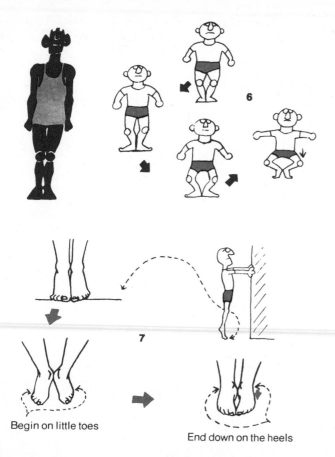

Bowed legs or pigeon toes

When standing erect, it is normal for there to be a slight opening between the thighs, knees, and ankles, but if this opening is larger than the width of two fingers, a conscious effort is required to correct it.

6. With thighs, calves, and heels as close together as possible, turn toes out so that feet make one straight line. Raise heels and do deep knee bends.

Flat feet

There are many ways to correct flat feet, such as standing on a broom handle or wearing an arch support in one's shoes. An even better suggestion involves the following exercise:

7. Stand on tiptoe with feet together, holding on to something to keep balance. Let yourself slowly down to your heels by way of the outsides of your feet, so that first the bases of the little toes touch, then the heels.

6

7

Begin on little toes

End down on the heels

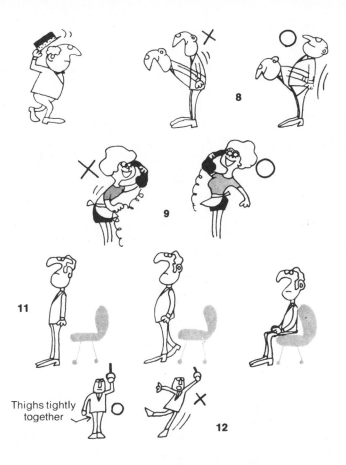

Thighs tightly together →

Reminders for good posture

Good posture is a matter of habit. Below are nine key points you should always remember.

8. After bowing, stand perfectly erect.

9. Stand perfectly erect when talking on the phone.

10. Walk with the chest broadened and the hips thrust slightly forward.

11. To sit down, stand facing forward in front of the chair, move one leg backward until it touches the front edge of the chair, sit down, and then draw your legs together. Always sit with back erect.

12. Learn the habit of keeping your balance when standing on the bus or train by tensing your inner thigh muscles.

13. Always counteract the effect of working in a hunched-over position by doing some form of back-bending exercise.

14. Keep good posture when doing warm-ups or cooling-down exercises.

15. If you have weak leg, torso, or back muscles, no matter how much attention you pay to posture, it will do no good. You must keep up your daily exercises.

16. Take heed of the proverb: "One man's fault is another man's lesson." An awareness of the posture of others will make you more aware of your own.

If you devote just one month of conscious effort to improving your posture, the results will be clear and rewarding, and you will come to understand the wisdom in the words of Musashi quoted at the beginning of this chapter.

59

Chapter 12. Preventing Back Problems

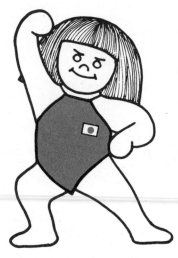

Heart disease, which results in part from lack of physical exercise, is popularly known in Japan as the "civilization disease." Another disease of civilization which has gained wide attention is lumbago, or back pain. This also is a result of lack of exercise, in particular, exercise of the legs, and ranks foremost among the problems with which company health counselors deal.

Of course, there is a variety of back problems and a variety of causes. An athlete may develop back pain from overwork of the back muscles, but the most common cause today is lack of exercise. When leg strength declines, there is a corresponding decline in the back muscles. This weakness leaves the individual highly vulnerable to unexpected pain from the slightest overexertion or from an unusual body position. A medical survey taken at a certain company showed that almost seventy percent of the employees had suffered at one time or another from back pain.

This chapter will explore ways to prevent back problems.

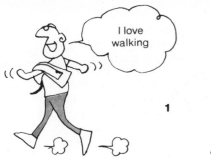
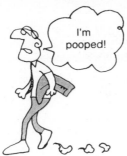

Legwork

If you have a bad back, idly stretching it or pounding it with your fists will solve no problems. You have got to begin where the problem itself begins—with the legs. People support on two legs what originally was meant to be supported by four. Therefore, to do the huge task assigned to them, the legs need to be in good condition. But the unfortunate reality of our modern age is that the legs receive increasingly less exercise. Walking, a lot of walking, is the most natural exercise for the legs (**1**), but everything in our rushed, mechanistic society mitigates against this. The inevitable result is widespread back pain.

Correct posture

Walking is a good cure for back pain, but bad posture will negate any good that walking might do. Since World War II, our school system has neglected this crucial aspect of education, and the people suffer as a result. It is thus important to heighten the consciousness of each individual in his posture, both at work and when walking. The two things to remember are to walk with the hips rather than with the legs, and to thrust the lower trunk forward, keeping it high as you walk (**2**).

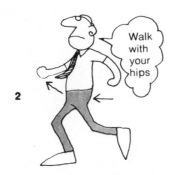

Do preventive exercises every day

Fatigue often settles in the lower back, leaving one feeling lethargic and heavy. When this gets unbearable, we pound our back with our fists, rotate the hips in an effort to relieve the pain, or have someone massage us. And when we have stiff shoulders we do the same, trying to relieve the stiffness with stretching and massage.

Below are some preventive exercises which you should do regularly at the specified times each day, one minute apiece in the morning before brushing your teeth, at noon, and before bed at night. The morning and evening exercises are different each day. *The noon exercise is always the same.*

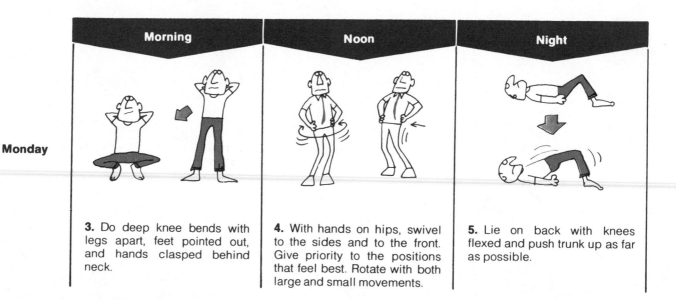

Monday

Morning

3. Do deep knee bends with legs apart, feet pointed out, and hands clasped behind neck.

Noon

4. With hands on hips, swivel to the sides and to the front. Give priority to the positions that feel best. Rotate with both large and small movements.

Night

5. Lie on back with knees flexed and push trunk up as far as possible.

Morning

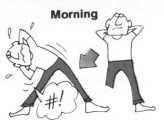

6. With hands clasped behind neck and legs spread, bend at the waist and try to touch elbows to knees 2 times right and left.

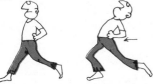

8. Thrust one leg forward, and arch back with hands supporting lower back.

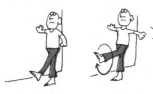

10. Stand on one leg, keeping balance with one hand on the wall, and swing free leg in circles in front of you.

Noon

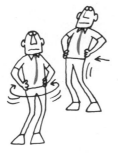

Night

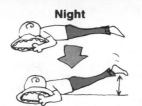

7. Lying on your stomach, with pillow beneath face, lift both legs together as high as possible.

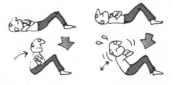

9. Do sit-ups with arms across chest and knees flexed. If this is difficult, sit up as far as you can.

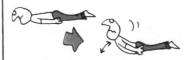

11. Lie on stomach and lift head and shoulders as far as possible.

Tuesday

Wednesday

Thursday

63

Friday

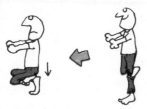

12. Stand on one leg, with the other folded around behind the knee. Squat, as if sitting in a chair, and return to standing position.

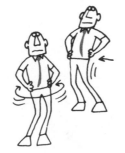

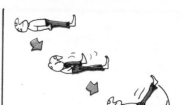

13. Lie on back and pull one knee tightly to chest. Then release, straighten and lift leg, and return it to floor.

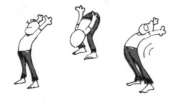

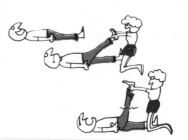

Saturday

14. Stand with legs spread and arms raised overhead. Bend at waist and let arms and upper body fall naturally forward. Straighten up, and arch back.

15. Lie on back and have someone slowly raise your legs one at a time to at least a 90° angle.

Morning

Noon

Night

64

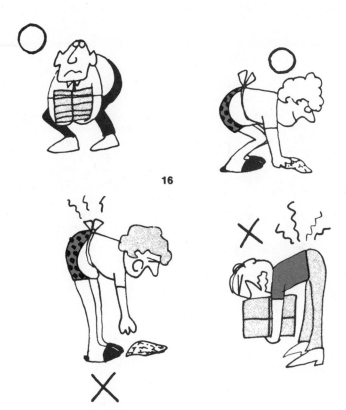

16

16. When picking something up or lifting a heavy object, always use your knees rather than your back. Thoughtlessly picking something up with the knees straight is the biggest immediate cause of back injuries. Working in a standing position with the back leaning even slightly forward is also a source of undue stress.

Of course, one should always consult a doctor about persistent or serious back problems, but if one observes the above caution and faithfully performs the preventive exercises each day, he or she will be free of pain and discomfort.

Chapter 13. Walking

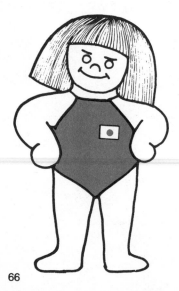

Everyone knows how to walk, but whether everyone knows how to walk *well* is another matter. To begin with, how many people have ever thought about how they walk? The human body was originally meant to walk on four legs rather than two. And despite the extraordinary stress which as a result is placed on the back and legs, the conveniences of modern life leave us increasingly weak and thus susceptible to back problems. Behind this all, however, there lurks the persistent problem of posture discussed previously. And, as we have seen, posture is all but neglected in most physical fitness programs.

One of the most physically fit figures in premodern Japan was the *ninja,* that agile black-clothed spy seen so often in samurai movies and television dramas **(1)**. It is said that the *ninja* had a repertoire of ten different styles of walking from which he would choose the style appropriate to each situation. Basic training for the *ninja,* however, consisted in the simple, yet difficult matter of walking a straight line, and toward this end, he would practice on a length of rope stretched on the ground.

Undoubtedly, there is a lesson in this for us, but we must begin at the even more fundamental level of consciousness. We must assume at the outset that our style of walking is awkward and inefficient. Let us survey, for a moment, the variety of bad walking habits common around us. See if you recognize yourself in any of them.

Most common among Japanese women is the stooped-shoulder walk, with face turned slightly downward **(2)**. Among men, it is the Charlie Chaplin duckfooted walk **(3)**. But there also is the pigeon-toed knock-kneed walk **(4)** and the hip-swinging "rumba" **(5)**. There are the bouncers and there are those who kick their legs back as they walk, some inward, others outward **(6)**.

The *ninja* is an extreme case, but even the common people in traditional Japan had a certain way for walking quickly on flat ground and another for walking long distances without getting tired. They had a way for walking up hills and a way for walking down. The great attention paid in traditional Japan to style in walking and other physical movement stands in marked contrast to the modern lack of concern about such things. We would profit by considering the example of the past.

The only distinctions modern Japanese make are between slow and fast gaits, large and small strides, and of course, good and bad posture. However, when basic physical fitness falls into a decline, we fail to make even these distinctions. The rest of this chapter will examine the matter of walking in greater detail.

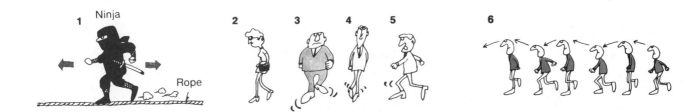

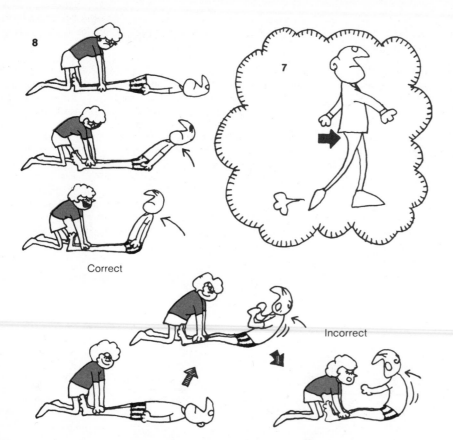

Correct

Incorrect

Walk with the hips

It may sound strange, but if we have it fixed in mind that we walk with the legs, we tire much more readily. Our legs begin to drag, our knees don't straighten out fully, and we lose the centeredness of a good walking posture.

If on the other hand we walk with our hips, thrusting the lower trunk slightly forward so that the back is perfectly straight, the chest will seem more expansive and we will cut a smart figure as we walk down the street **(7).**

Strengthen the back

Good posture is 80 percent of walking well. To improve posture, do the following exercises every day:

8. Sit-ups: At first, have someone hold your ankles or knees. Arch your back as you sit up to exercise the back muscles. Rounded-back sit-ups strengthen stomach muscles, but it is the back muscles which need strengthening for good posture.

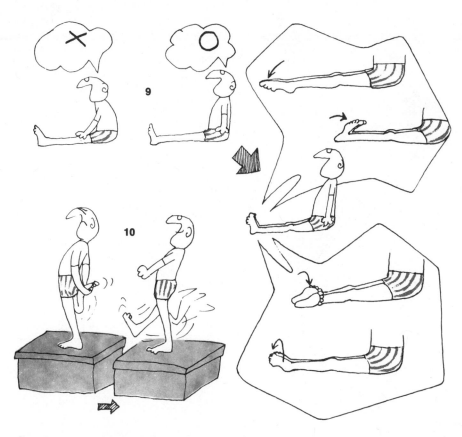

9. Ankle exercise: Sit on the floor with the legs stretched out. Make sure that back is not slumped, that shoulders are not stooped, and that head is not tilted forward. Relax shoulders and point toes forward, backward, and to the left and right. Do this rhythmically for one minute without losing posture.

10. Leg relaxation: Stand on one leg, holding the other behind by the ankle with both hands. Do a brief isometric exercise, forcing down with the leg. Then release all tension from the leg and let it fall naturally. Do this 5 times with both legs. You may find it easier to do on a low platform.

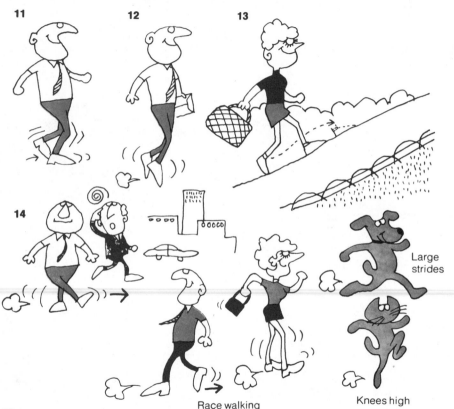

11

12

13

14

Large strides

Race walking

Knees high

Be aware of various walking styles

Above all, it is important first to be *aware* of how we walk. In part, this is a matter of consciously noting the many ways in which others walk, perhaps even imitating them. This is not necessarily to acquire another's manner of walking, but rather to heighten awareness of one's own walk by physically contrasting it with that of others.

11. Put an occasional skip into your walk.

12. Twice a day, walk on tiptoe.

13. When walking a long distance, or even when walking up a hill, take long steps with one leg and shorter steps with the other, in the 6:4 ratio of the old walking manuals.

14. Practice walking sideways. It is not as easy as it seems. Cross one leg over and then stretch the other wide and quickly. Try not to turn shoulders.

The improvement of one's walking style means first correcting posture, which demands constant awareness and regular exercise. Posture is the basis not only of a good walking style but of physical fitness itself.

Chapter 14. Good-Morning Exercises

PART II. EXERCISES FOR EVERY DAY

Though our physical fitness campaign has made significant advances in recent years and there is widespread acceptance of the importance of regular exercise, persistent misconceptions remain. Many believe that the truly fit body is that of a body-builder. Others assume that exercising only once a week is sufficient. *It is yet to be universally understood that health and fitness are dependent upon a heightened awareness of our bodies and upon a daily regimen of exercise.* In order to help achieve this awareness, I have suggested many exercise programs which bring sports and exercising into the immediate circle of the individual's daily life. In each of the chapters in this part of the book, I will introduce a set of exercises for a particular moment of the day, beginning in this chapter with morning exercises.

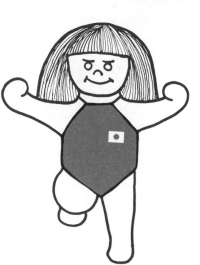

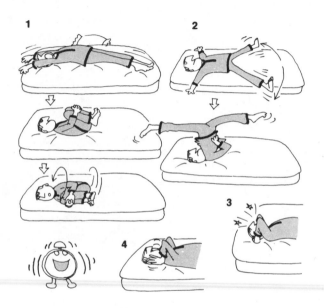

Late-night people are on the increase, and one trait they have in common is the habit of rushing off for work or school in the morning without properly washing or eating. This in effect is the same as throwing an engine into high gear without letting it warm up. No good can come of such a rash approach to living. For safety and a productive, healthy life, let us give our bodies the care they need and deserve. Let us turn the engine on early and give it a chance to warm up.

Eye-openers: exercises in bed

Do at least two of the following exercises for one minute every morning (increasing to two minutes as fitness improves).

1. After the initial stretch upon waking, clasp arms tightly around knees and roll to the right, to the left, then face up again and release legs.

2. With arms spread at sides, open and close legs, gradually increasing the distance until the inner thigh muscles almost begin to hurt. If you can, lift lower body into air, supporting back with hands, and spread legs to the front and back. This is a good way to beat a hangover.

3. Clasp arms behind neck and beat elbows lightly against head.

4. Rub face and neck with palms until warm. This is an age-old tried and tested measure for preserving the health and beauty of the skin.

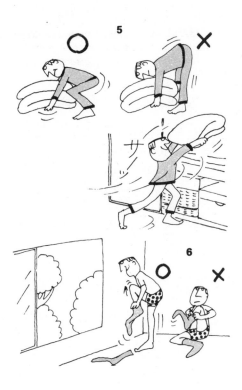

Dressing

Depending on the way you go about it, dressing and making the bed can serve as an exercise. Move briskly, bending at the knees to pick something up, rather than bending at the waist (**5**). Stand while dressing (**6**). Don't sit to put on footwear.

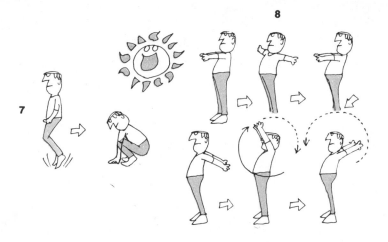

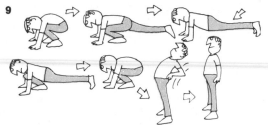

One-minute calisthenics

In your bedroom, in the hall, or in the yard, do some formal calisthenics before breakfast. Below are two possible series of quick exercises. Course A is for anyone; course B is for people in their twenties. Execute the forms of the exercises correctly and do the prescribed number of repetitions.

Course A for Everyone

7. Jump lightly twice and then squat. Do this 7 times.

8. Raise arms in front to shoulder height, spread to sides, and return to front. Then swing once in a full forward circle, and once in a full backward circle. Do this 7 times.

9. Crouch with palms on floor. Stretch right leg back and join it with left. Return right leg beneath buttocks, then left. Finally stand and arch back with hands on hips. Do this 7 times.

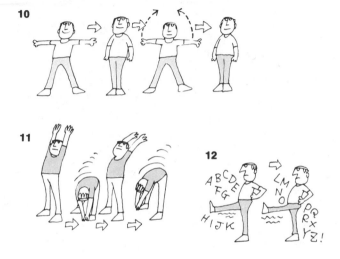

10. Jump and spread legs, at the same time raising arms to shoulder height, then jump again to the original arms-down position. Jump and spread legs again, this time raising arms overhead and clapping hands. Then jump back to original position. Do this 20 times.

11. With legs spread to shoulder width, stretch arms over head. Bend diagonally forward and touch fingers to right foot, rise up again, and bend to touch left foot. Do this 7 times.

12. With hands on hips, lift right leg, knee straight, and hold it while counting from A to K. Repeat with left leg, counting from L to Z.

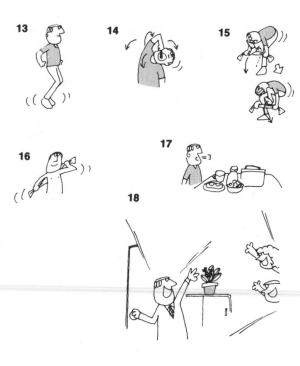

Quickie exercises

13. Jump 100 times up and down the hall or in the yard.

14. Stretch neck to sides, front, and back while brushing teeth. Do this 10 times.

15. After washing up, hold towel taut at both ends and step over it and back, one foot at a time. Do this 3 times left and right.

16. Rub naked upper body vigorously with a wet or dry towel for one minute.

17. Before beginning breakfast, do stomach breathing (see Chapter 22) for one minute.

18. As you leave the house, say "Goodbye" with a big healthy voice. Those who are seeing you off should answer likewise.

Chapter 15. Commuting

There are cynics who say that commuting to work during the rush hour is in itself enough to keep the body fit. On the face of it, this would hardly seem to be true, but it is possible to put commuting time to good use. In this chapter, I will suggest ways in which you can greatly increase the exercise potential of your traveling time.

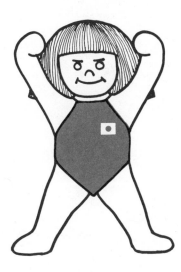

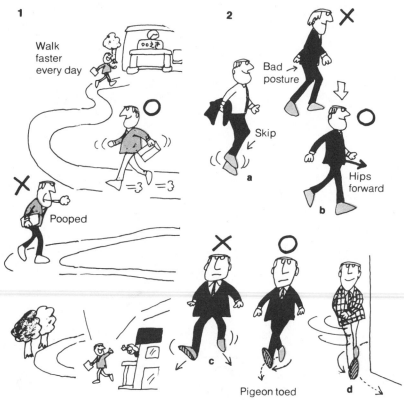

1

Walk faster every day

○

✗ Pooped

2

✗ Bad posture

Skip

a

=3 =3

○ Hips forward

b

✗ ○ Pigeon toed

c

d

Walking

Walking is a barometer of one's health, a way to slow the process of aging (in part because it is good for the blood circulation), and a good preparatory step to a more vigorous program of running.

1. Walk faster. If ordinarily it takes 15 minutes to walk to your station, do it in 14 minutes 30 seconds today, and tomorrow do it in 14 minutes.

2. If you watch, you will see that there are many different ways of walking. Most of them, unfortunately, are inefficient. Try a variety until you have found one that feels right to you. Below are some suggestions:

a) Put an occasional skip into your walk.

b) Walk with hips consciously thrust slightly forward.

c) Try walking slightly pigeon-toed.

d) When turning a corner, speed up slightly and cross outer foot over inner.

e) Occasionally exaggerate twisting of lower torso.

3. Keep an eye on the stoplights ahead and adjust pace so that you don't have to wait at any of them.

78

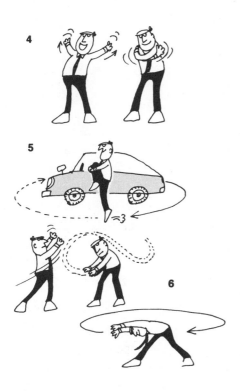

Driving

Before getting in car do the following three exercises:

4. Chest expansion and embracing: Spread arms wide and expand chest, then embrace yourself as tightly as possible. Do this 7 times.

5. Thigh-to-chest walking: Walk slowly around car, lifting knees high and pulling them to chest with arms.

6. Figure eights and torso rotation: With legs spread and a springiness in the knees, describe 6 figure eights in the air in front of you, using torso and arms together. For each figure eight, add a complete torso rotation. Do this 3 times to both right and left.

These three exercises, if done faithfully as a set each morning, will make you more alert at the wheel and will prevent back problems and weakening of the legs.

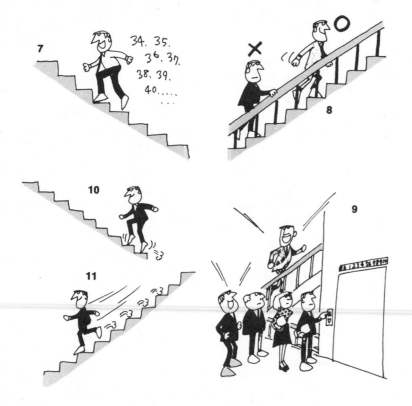

Ascending and descending stairs

7. Climb at least 100 steps per day (not counting descent). Most people have no idea even of how many steps they climb in their own train stations each working day of the year.

8. Do not use the handrail unless you are elderly or have a physical problem. It is particularly unbecoming for young persons to hold on to the rail.

9. Do not use escalator or elevator for up to three flights.

10. Ascend on tiptoe.

11. Sometimes descend as fast as you can. This will improve agility.

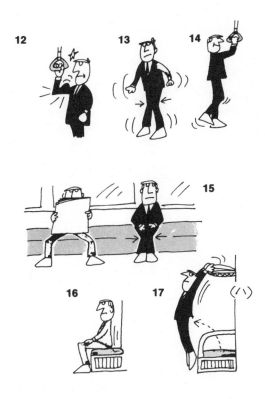

On public transportation

When standing

12. If you are holding on to a strap, see how long you can tense a muscle.

13. Practice keeping balance on moving vehicle by pressing thighs together.

14. Sometimes stand on one foot.

When sitting

15. Sit with legs together.

16. Occasionally stretch spine.

17. If you have placed a briefcase or something else light in the rack above where you are sitting, pick it up from behind your head without turning around.

As you can see, there are many exercises which one can do simply during the time it takes to go to work or school. And there are countless other variations. The essential elements, however, boil down to three: walk well and briskly, use the staircase whenever possible, and always maintain good posture. If you make a program as simple as this and stick to it, the difference in your health and general fitness will be clear after five or ten years.

Chapter 16. Noon at the Office

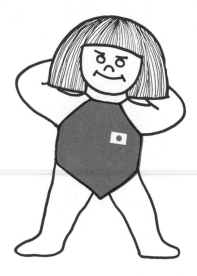

After lunch, many office workers go out for a cup of coffee, play *go* or *shōgi* (Japanese chess) in the office, or, if the weather is good, talk or nap on the lawn in front of their building. It seems that the common habit of lying around on holidays in front of the television set has been extended to the lunch break. This may be partly a result of the mistaken belief that one should not move around or exercise after eating. But if you consider that physical fitness is a round-the-clock matter, you will realize that even the free time after lunch is best used actively, rather than for passive rest. In this chapter, I will introduce the noon routines of two physical fitness enthusiasts.

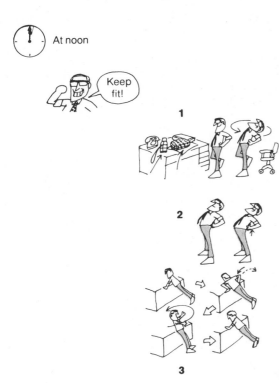

Mr. Narimatsu's Routine

Mr. Narimatsu is a department head in a downtown business firm. He is fifty-one, but around his office he is known as "Mr. Physical Fitness" because of his trim build and muscle tone. Ten years ago, however, he was overweight and concerned about his dangerously high blood pressure. On the advice of his doctor he started an exercise program, for which he kept a training suit and running shoes in his locker at the office.

Exercises at noon

He does these for 2 minutes before lunch:

1. Standing on one leg with hands on hips, he slowly rotates his neck from side to side. Then he repeats this standing on other leg.

2. Back bends: With hands at lower back and thumbs pressing hard against the muscles bordering the spine, he arches back. He then straightens up, raises the position of his thumbs slightly, and arches back again. He applies pressure longest where it feels best, because the muscles there are the tightest.

3. Diagonal push-up position body-twists: In a diagonal push-up position with hands on the edge of his desk, he bends arms, pushes himself strongly up, and twists in the air, landing again on hands. He does this alternately to the right and left.

At 12:30

4

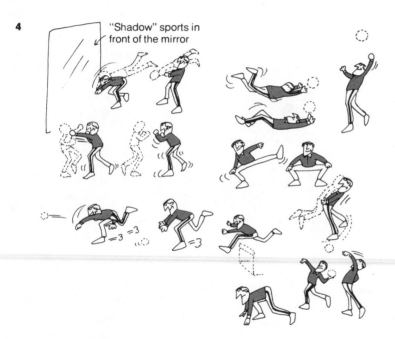

"Shadow" sports in front of the mirror

Exercises at 12:30

After a lunch of vegetable juice and a sandwich, Mr. Narimatsu rests for a short while and then changes into his training suit for a quick workout in the company's gym.

4. Mirror boxing: For warm-ups, he goes through the basic motions of a variety of sports in front of a large mirror. Each day he does a different sport, such as judo throws; jab, straight, and uppercut in boxing; tumbling return and spike serve in volleyball; pitching and fielding in baseball; shoulder throw and overhand throw in sumo; hurdles, discus, shot-put, and racing start in track and field.

5

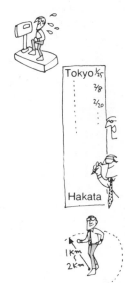

Tokyo 1/25
7/8
2/20

Hakata

1 Km
2 Km

5. Running machine: Mr. Narimatsu tries to run the equivalent of 2 km (1.2 miles) each lunch period on the running machine. He keeps track of his total distance on a chart which lists the stations on the bullet train from Tokyo to Hakata. His goal this year is to reach Kyoto. Mr. Narimatsu is also interested in local history, so when the weather is good, he leaves the building to jog to some significant site within a 2-km (1.2-mile) radius. On occasion, he even goes as far as 4 km (2.4 miles) away, returning for lack of time on a bus or subway. After about 20 minutes of exercising, he showers and plunges back refreshed into his work. The energy he exudes affects his whole department in a positive way. That more than anything is the reason why Mr. Narimatsu is so satisfied with his exercise program.

Mr. Ueno's Health Routine

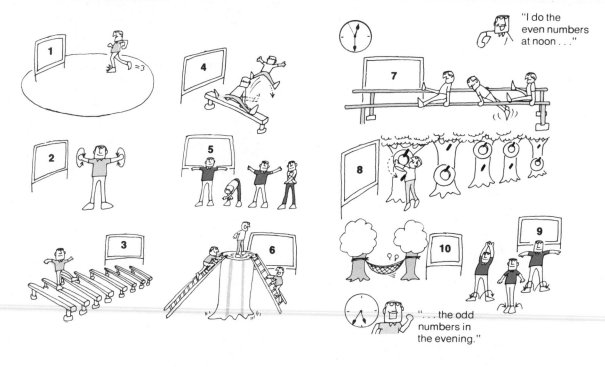

"I do the even numbers at noon . . ."

". . . the odd numbers in the evening."

Mr. Ueno's Routine

Mr. Ueno is forty and works as an outdoor supervisor in a manufacturing plant. His factory covers a large area which has a gymnasium, a playing field, and tennis courts, as well as a health walk. Mr. Ueno uses the health walk for his exercise program. During his lunch hour he exercises at the even-numbered stops along it, and after work, at the odd-numbered stops. If it rains, he wears a raincoat.

1. Achilles-tendon stretching   10 revolutions.
2. Arm rotating   10 times, both forward and backward.
3. Log walking.
4. Open-legged log vaulting   5 times.
5. Arm-swinging forward bends   10 times.
6. Ladder climbing   3 times.
7. Legs-up parallel-bar crossing.
8. Tire hanging   10 times.
9. Double jumping-jacks 10 times.
10. Hammock rest   3 minutes.

Chapter 17. Noon at Home

Some people have lunch at the same time every day. Others eat at different times. Each group needs a different exercise schedule. In this chapter, I will outline a noon exercise program for the person at home who organizes her morning in the usual fashion—breakfast cleanup, housecleaning, laundry, and then preparation for lunch.

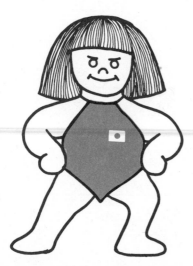

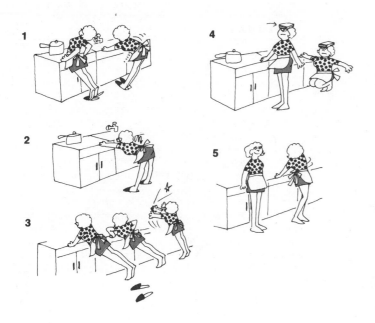

In the kitchen

Exercises using the kitchen counter

1. Back arching and stomach contractions: Work around the house involves much bending over. As an antidote, stand on tiptoe in front of the counter and, while waiting for the kettle to boil or whatever, pull against the counter and arch back. Then straighten arms, rock onto heels, curve back, and contract stomach. Repeat slowly and deliberately.

2. Back stretching: Place hands at shoulder width on the counter and bend forward at the waist until arms and back are in one straight line.

3. Diagonal hand-clap push-ups: Lean forward and place hands at shoulder width on the counter so that arms and torso are at a 90° angle. Bend elbows to let yourself down, and straighten them strongly to push yourself up and clap hands. This is a good exercise to get rid of excess fat on the upper arm.

4. Deep knee bends: Stand sideways with one hand on counter as in ballet class and, balancing a book on head, do slow deep knee bends.

5. Torso twisting: Stand with back to counter and feet together. Slowly twist sideways without shifting feet and place both hands on counter. At first stand close to counter and use momentum to swing yourself around, but gradually move away and touch it from a distance.

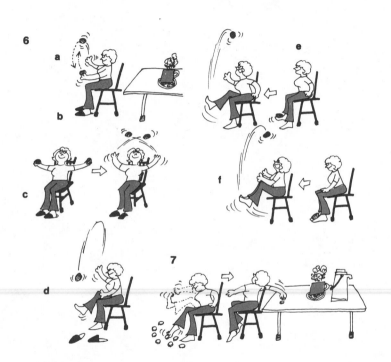

6. Using beanbags: The beanbag is usually thought of as a child's toy, but it also can be a useful piece of exercise equipment for the housewife.

a) Juggle two beanbags, one in each hand. Toss beanbag from right hand into air, and before catching it in left, pass other beanbag in left hand to right.

b) Do above in the reverse order, starting with left hand.

c) Hold arms out at sides with a beanbag in each hand, throw beanbags simultaneously over head, and catch them in opposite hands.

d) Toss one beanbag at a time into air and catch it on top of foot.

e) Place beanbag on foot, toss it in air by lifting thighs, and catch it with one hand.

f) Do above with one beanbag on each foot.

7. Bottle-top pickup: Place a number of bottle tops at feet and pick them up one at a time with the toes of one foot, passing them as fast as possible to hand and then to counter. Then use the other foot. You might also try the same exercise using single sheets of newspaper.

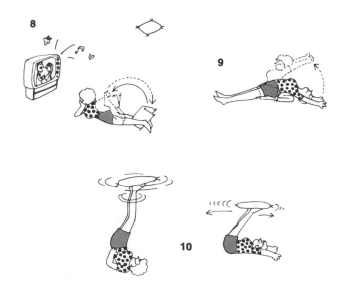

While watching television

The average amount of time that people watch television at home is increasing. Many, for example, watch while eating lunch. Of course, it would be impossible to exercise, eat, and watch television all at once, but after lunch you can rest in front of the TV screen and get some light exercise at the same time.
On tatami (straw mats) or a rug using a cushion

8. While lying on stomach, chin propped up with hands, hold a folded cushion firmly between ankles. Bending at knees, slowly raise it to touch your back and return it to floor. During commercials, you can do this exercise faster and lose excess fat from thighs.

9. During commercials, fold cushion in two or three, place it under small of back, and rest with eyes closed. When the program starts again, raise yourself in a slow sit-up. You may not be able to do this at first, but when you can, you will know that you are on the way to becoming fit.

10. During commercials, lie face up with knees flexed and a cushion between feet. Bring cushion as close to face as possible, or stretch legs so it is as far away as possible. Sometimes, lift waist and legs straight into air, with support from hands at lower back, and balance cushion on top of feet. This exercise is surprisingly effective in reviving one's spirits.

In a chair, using a 1-m (1-yard) elastic string

11. Hold the elastic string at both ends and stretch across chest by extending arms to sides. Later, use two or three strands at once.

12. Place string around neck and pull forward with arms, backward with neck.

13. Lift knees up and place string around bottoms of feet. As you pull back on string, slowly stretch legs out. Repeat, as if rowing a boat.

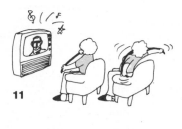

11

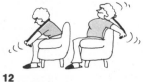

12

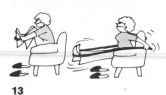

13

Chapter 18. Midafternoon

By 3:00, the busy person is ready for a rest. A large part of the day's work is done, but there is still much left to be finished. With good reason, many Japanese offices choose this time for group calisthenics. Rather than quietly sipping a cup of tea or coffee, it is much healthier to be physically active. Exercise helps dispel fatigue and provides a change of pace which allows one to return to work with renewed interest and vigor.

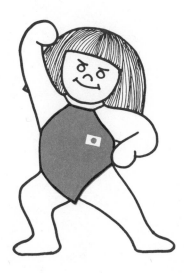

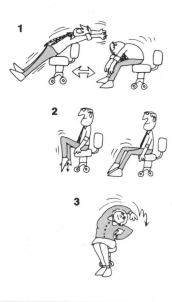

At the office (while seated)

1. Full back stretches: As if to yawn, stretch arms behind head and stretch legs straight out. Then slump forward, letting arms hang loosely in front. Do this 2 times.

2. Heel lifts: Alternately lift right and left heels as high as possible, with toes on floor. Do this 20 times with feet near chair and 20 times with legs somewhat extended.

3. Side bends: Sitting erect and with left hand tucked under arm, throw right hand over head to the left and bend at the waist. Repeat to the right. Do this 2 times left and 2 times right.

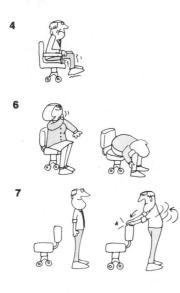

4. Body lifts: Raise yourself in a seated position from chair for 5 to 10 seconds.

5. Neck bends and rotation: With eyes closed, bend neck to sides, back, and front. Then rotate it first to the left, then to the right.

6. Shoulder, arm, and leg massage: With right hand, massage left shoulder, arm, elbow, and the gaps between fingers on the left hand. Repeat with left hand on right side. Finally, bend over and massage legs, thighs, and calves. Concentrate on spots where it feels best.

7. Torso twisting: Stand with back to chair 50 cm (20 inches) away, and spread legs to shoulder width. Slowly twist torso to right and place hands on back of chair. Repeat to left. Do this 3 times in each direction.

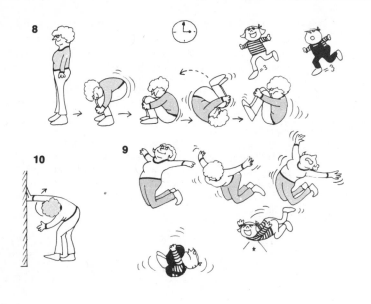

At home

From late afternoon through evening, the woman at home is busy with shopping, various household chores, supper preparations, and dishwashing. Before beginning this last part of her day, she can benefit from the following exercises.

8. Get small, get big: From a standing position, crouch down with rounded back and clasp knees. Sit, and without loosening hold around knees, roll backward. Use reflexive momentum to get back to feet. Stand erect and stretch arms high over head.

9. Torso tilting: Kneel erect with arms raised at sides. Tilt from waist as far forward as possible without falling, stretching arms backward to keep balance. Do the same to the sides and diagonally to the rear.

10. Ducking: Stand with the palm of right hand planted flat against a wall or doorway. Without moving hand, duck under arm, left arm leading the way. Then place left palm against wall and duck under with right arm leading the way. Gradually lower the position of the hand on the wall, seeing how far down and how fast you can duck. Since you are alternating turns to the right and left, there is no reason why you should become dizzy, but if you do, slow the pace. Do this 10 times both left and right.

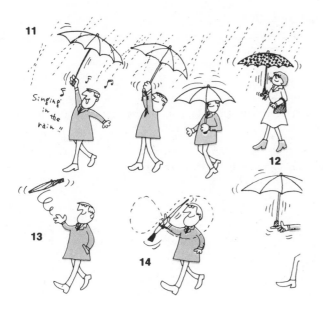

In the rain

Not only in midafternoon but at any time of day when you are walking in the rain, you can do the following umbrella exercises.

11. Hold umbrella high with outstretched arm. Then raise free hand, take umbrella into it, and hold it low.

12. Balance umbrella on one or two fingers.

13. If rain has let up and you are carrying a collapsible umbrella, toss and spin it in the air as you walk. Or, if it is a long umbrella, extend it with one hand around back, give it a light toss, and see if you can catch it with the same hand on the other side.

14. Holding umbrella in the middle, twirl it in sideways figure eights, like a baton twirler. You must be careful, of course, not to poke anyone.

Chapter 19. In the Bath and Before Supper

It has always been Mr. Hamada's custom to take a bath with his son before supper each evening. The Japanese bathroom, unlike American bathrooms, is meant solely for bathing; the toilet is in a separate room. The floor of the Japanese bathroom is covered with tile and fitted with a drain so that one can wash and rinse outside of the tub, leaving the bathwater clean for leisurely soaking. It is not at all uncommon for several members of a family to bathe together, as do the Hamadas. For 5 minutes before taking their bath, Mr. Hamada and his son do the following exercises.

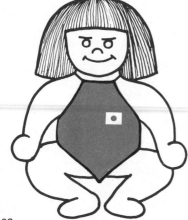

Pre-bath exercises for two

1. Foot stomping: Hold hands while facing each other, and try to step on each other's feet. The first to do this 5 times is the winner.

2. Catch and roll: Sit facing with legs spread, and pass a rolled bath towel back and forth. Catch the towel high and roll over backward, bringing legs overhead and using the towel for a pillow. When you return the pass, aim so that the partner can catch it easily above his head.

3. Towel pull: There are many variants on this exercise. One is for the father to lie on his back and hold the towel between his feet while the child pulls at the other end. Another is to put a floor cushion on top of one end of the towel and have the child try to put the father off-balance by pulling the other end. The child will like this exercise.

Before getting in the water

4. Weigh yourself and mark your weight down on a chart.

5. Expand chest with arms stretched over head. Then, in a relaxed position, with feet spread at shoulder width, clasp hands behind buttocks and slowly raise them up back. Arch head back and expand chest. Feel the rightness of good posture.

6. Crouch as low as possible, with legs spread and hands on knees, like a sumo wrestler facing his opponent at the beginning of a match.

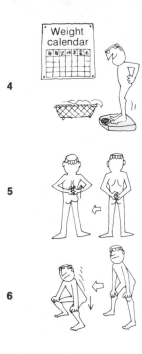

4

5

6

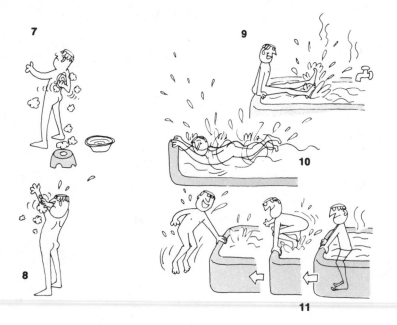

When soaping down

7. Wash from head to toe with just one hand or the other, scrubbing even the hard-to-reach back. This will help prevent stiffening shoulders in middle age.

8. After washing once with a cloth and rinsing off, soap down again and massage whole body with bare hands.

In the tub

9. Sit on edge of tub and exercise lower legs as if doing the backstroke. Be careful not to tip over.

10. If tub is long enough, turn onto stomach and vigorously exercise entire body.

11. When leaving the tub (if you are under forty), vault out in one clean movement.

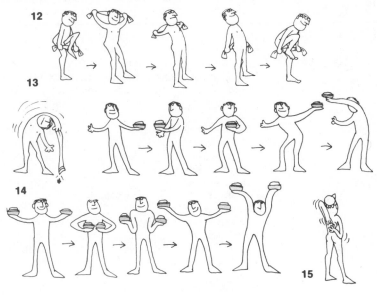

Not only is the Japanese bath separate from the toilet, it is also separate from, though adjacent to, a dressing room.

12. Dry yourself vigorously by holding towel taut at both ends.

13. Does towel touch floor when you hold it over head and bend to the side?

14. Can you hold a soap dish in the palm of one hand and do the maneuvers shown in the illustrations? How about with a soap dish in each hand?

15. Can you touch fingers behind back as shown in the drawing?

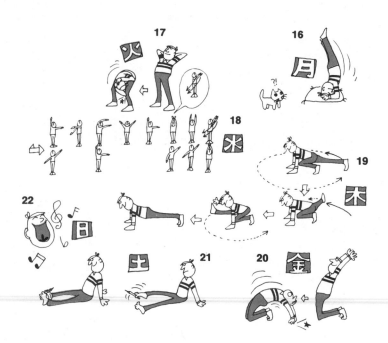

Before supper

A young student called for supper will often stand up from his desk and stretch once before going downstairs. Why not incorporate something into your daily routine just as simple as that yawn and stretch, but with more exercise potential? This is particularly important for junior high and high school students who study so hard and get so little exercise. Here is one week's worth of suggestions.

16. Monday: Stand on head, placing elbows in a triangular relationship to head for balance. Lift legs slowly so as not to tumble over backward. Hold for 5 seconds.

17. Tuesday: Stand with legs at shoulder width, hands clasped behind neck and elbows spread wide. Alternately touch left elbow to right knee and right elbow to left knee. Do this 10 times both left and right.

18. Wednesday: Spell out some simple phrase such as "Today was a beautiful day," using semaphore signals.

19. Thursday: Crouch down with palms on floor and extend right leg back. Circle extended leg twice counterclockwise, then twice clockwise. Do the same with left leg, first clockwise, then counterclockwise.

20. Friday: Kneel erect with arms stretched over head. Bend over backward until fingers touch floor, and return to upright position.

21. Saturday: Sitting on floor, pick up a pencil with toes of right foot and pass it to left foot.

22. Sunday: Take a deep breath and sing in a low range, "do, re, mi, fa, so, la, ti, do" in 10 seconds. Repeat in a high range. Then do the same in both low and high ranges, this time taking 15 seconds for each.

Chapter 20. After-Dinner Exercises for Fun

The evening hours, after the supper dishes have been washed, are a time for reading, watching television, sipping tea, and talking. But even during this time, there are exercises which you can enjoy.

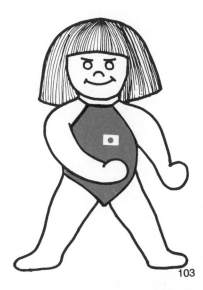

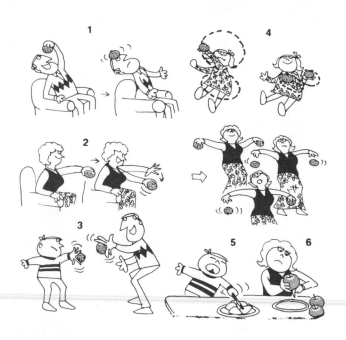

Dessert-time exercises

1. Tangerine balancing: Balance a tangerine on forehead. See if you can roll it back and forth on forehead by moving neck slightly.

2. Tangerine drop and catch: Hold tangerine at shoulder level with outstretched arm. Let it go, and catch it with same hand before it falls to floor. Make it your goal to catch it 4 out of 5 times. Also try with tangerines in both hands. These exercises are good for the reflexes.

3. Finger spreading: Hold tangerine between two adjacent fingers (pointing and middle fingers, or middle and ring fingers).

4. Sit on floor and describe figure eights with tangerine resting in palm of hand. This is easy enough when doing horizontal figure eights, but you may find it more difficult to do vertical ones, having to twist both arm and torso.

5. Eyes-closed forking: Choose an apple or persimmon section and see if you can stab it, eyes closed, with a fork or toothpick.

6. Backward peeling: Many can peel an apple or persimmon from the top down in one continuous peel. But how many can do it from the bottom up?

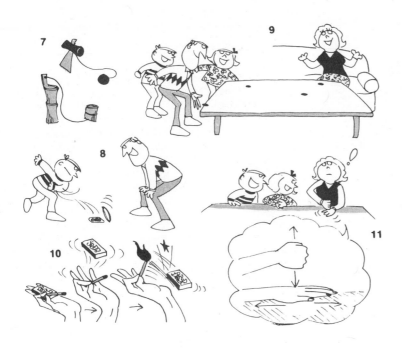

Games

The evening is a good time for traditional indoor games such as cup and ball, cat's cradle, and paper cutting.

7. Cup and ball: The traditional cup-and-ball set has been replaced by modern commercial versions, but you will find it easy and rewarding to make your own. Simply cut a section of bamboo for a ball and another slightly larger section to catch it in, and tie these two together.

8. Ringtoss is an enjoyable indoor game.

9. Coin shooting: Quarters are placed so that they extend slightly beyond the edge of a table. Each person hits his coin with the palm of his hand, making it slide as far as possible without going over the other side.

10. One-handed match lighting: With one hand remove match from box and hold it between thumb and pointing finger, with box resting on other three fingers. Flip box into air and strike match against it as it falls.

11. Coordination test: Place both hands on table, the right one closed in a fist and the left open, with palm faced down. As you rub open palm against table, move fist up and down. When you have both hands moving correctly, change so that left hand is moving up and down in a fist and right hand is rubbing table in an open palm.

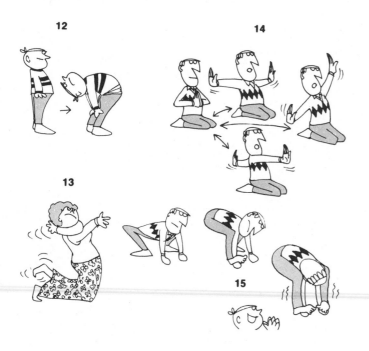

Traditional calisthenics

Here are some exercises that Japanese did before Western influences arrived in the late nineteenth century.

12. Back-of-knee touching: Stand with legs together and arch back to grasp the backs of knees.

13. Ear touching: Balance on knees with one foot lifted. Wrap right arm all the way around neck and touch right ear. Do opposite with left arm. Then simultaneously touch left ear with right hand and right ear with left hand.

14. Arm stretching: Kneel in formal position, with rump on heels. Place hands together as if praying. Slowly stretch arms, palms out, to the sides, then return to the praying position. Repeat diagonally to the sides, then to the front and back. Inhale as you stretch arms out, and exhale as you return them to the praying position.

15. Feet on fists: Crouch down and set fists on floor, as a sumo wrestler does when he faces his opponent at the beginning of a match. Place arch of left foot on left fist. Then place arch of right foot on right fist. Finally, stand on both fists at once.

Chapter 21. At Bedtime

Throughout the day and throughout the year, one should be alert to the constant need for exercise and be aware of the infinite number of ways in which this need can easily and readily be met. With this chapter we reach the last set of exercises for a particular moment of the day.

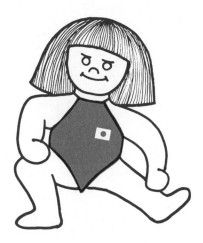

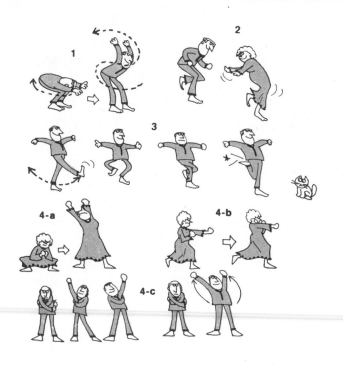

Tension-releasing exercises

When one changes for the night, one casts off all the cares and trials of the day. Dressed in lightweight, loose-fitting nightwear, one can be relaxed in a way one couldn't be even during the family hour between supper and bedtime. This special feeling of release can be given expression in the following exercises.

1. Rising body swing: In this variation of stretching, start in a crouching position, with head down and arms forward. Rise slowly, swinging arms and torso in an S-shape. Do 2, 3, or more of these depending on your mood.

2. The twist: Twist and turn as if dancing to rock music. This is good for a torso and chest which have been locked into the staid routines of daily life.

3. Foot swinging: Stand on one leg. Swing other leg freely back and forth, turn it and swing it to the sides, wrap it behind standing leg, or kick it back and up from the knee to strike rump.

4. Martial arts cheerleading exercises:

a) Touching the heavens: With legs spread wide and fists brought together in front of chest, sink to a crouching position. Rise up, stretch arms forcefully into air, and tilt head toward ceiling.

b) Forward arm thrusts: Open legs fore and back, make fists, and thrust arms alternately forward. The forward fist should be facing downward, while the retracted fist should be facing upward. A variation of this is to have the extended hand open though still facing downward, and the retracted hand closed in an upward fist.

c) Stand with feet spread and arms wrapped tight across chest. Raise arms alternately or together.

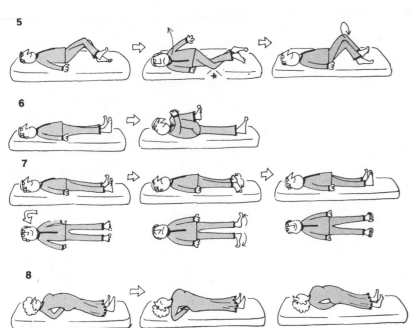

Sleep-tight exercises

5. Hip twists: Lie on back with one knee flexed and the other crossed over it. In that position, roll slowly over and touch knee to bed.

6. Knee to chest: Lying on back, bring knees one at a time to chest, holding knee firm with arms, and return it slowly to bed. Do this 2 times.

7. Foot exercise: Lie on back with feet pointing straight up. Turn feet outward as far as possible. Point feet back up again, and then point them forward as if to press them down on bed. Do this 2 times.

8. Self back massage: Make fists and place them beneath back so that knuckles are pressed against muscles which border spine. Move gradually up and down spine, holding fists 3 seconds at each place, or 5 to 10 seconds in places where it feels particularly good.

9. Buttocks press: Remaining on back, press both thumbs as hard as possible against the concave sides of the buttocks. If this hurts, it is an indication of tension. Further pressing will bring some relief.

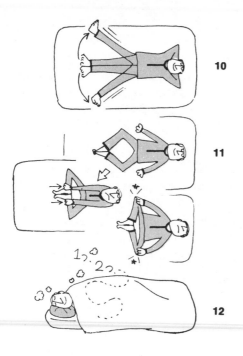

10. Leg spreading: Slowly open and close legs while lying on back with hands behind head. If you know how far you can usually spread them, this will serve as a measure of how stiff your thighs are.

11. Frog legs: Place bottoms of feet together and pull up with hands. In that position, press knees down to bed as far as possible.

12. Self-hypnosis: The best sleeping posture, at least while falling asleep, is on the back with arms and legs spread slightly. Pull covers up. Close eyes and count breaths. Imagine a clear blue sky, and feel yourself slowly sinking into the softness of the bed. You are tired. Sleep well. If you have trouble breathing or if your stomach is uneasy, lie on the right side.

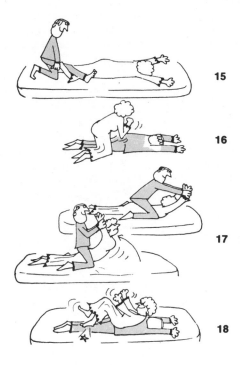

15

16

17

18

Sleep-tight exercises for couples

If you sleep with a mate, you might try the following exercises together.

13. Bridge: One partner arches back to make a bridge. The other crawls under and supports for 30 seconds. Reverse and repeat.

14. Palms together: Face each other in push-up position. While holding yourself up with one hand, put the other hand together with partner's. Alternate hands rhythmically, perhaps while singing a song.

Sleep-tight massage for couples

15. Leg presses: One partner lies face down. The other extends calf of right leg over partner's right knee, lifts partner's lower leg from the ankle, and presses it against his own. Repeat with other leg.

16. Elbow massage: One partner massages rump and lower back of other with elbows. If you find a spot which is particularly tense and sensitive, soften it

17. Back arching: One partner lies face down. The other kneels on top, picks partner up by forearms, and slowly arches back.

18. Back-on-back leg massage: One partner lies face down. The other lies face up on top and gently massages partner's legs with feet.

Chapter 22. Preventing Sleeplessness

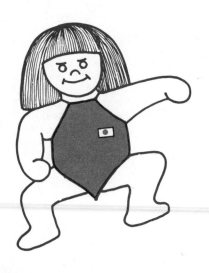

What could be worse than hunger when there is no food to eat? There are those who would answer that sleeplessness when there is no sleep is just as bad if not worse, for sleeplessness is indeed a kind of hunger. And it can be even more frustrating if beside you, or in the next room, you can hear the peaceful breathing or snoring of someone who is sound asleep. That irritation itself can be an impediment to sleep.

Everyone has had difficulty in falling asleep at one time or another, either because of nervous tension from overwork, drinking coffee or strong tea, or some other stimulation. Such occurrences, however, do not often interrupt normal life. They are infrequent and usually result in deep sleep the following night. And if a person has difficulty sleeping the first night in an unfamiliar bed, he or she adjusts to it quickly enough to be back on a regular schedule by the next night.

And quite often, people who complain that they couldn't sleep have actually had quite enough sleep. At least, they have slept a sufficient number of hours. Their problem is that they haven't slept deeply enough.

Nevertheless, insomnia is a severe problem for some, more so now in our complex modern world than it once was. Such people become caught in a vicious cycle of sleeplessness and the use of sleep-inducing drugs, which can damage the heart and blood vessels.

In this chapter, I will discuss ways to prevent insomnia through exercise and modified sleeping habits.

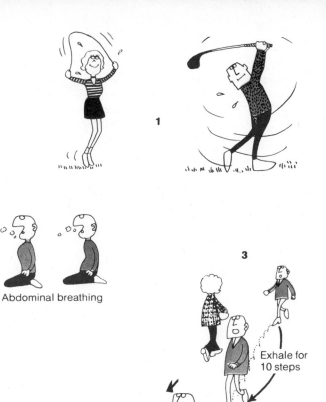

1

2

Abdominal breathing

3

Exhale for
10 steps

Exhale for
10 steps

Inhale for
1 step

Exercise at least 15 minutes a day

Insomnia can be considered the result of a lop-sided rhythm of activity and rest in a person's life. At work, at home, or at a sports club, become involved in some form of sport or exercise **(1)**.

Learn abdominal breathing

Together with indifference toward posture, our physical education suffers from a lack of interest in the art of breathing. This is unfortunate, since breathing control is one of the central pillars of such Eastern systems of exercise and meditation as Indian yoga and Chinese *dōin*. These systems are important to us today because they emphasize the improved functioning of internal organs for outward effect.

Ordinarily, we expand the chest to inhale. This is called chest breathing. Of course, it keeps us alive, but there is another type of breathing, called abdominal breathing, which, if practiced regularly, can bring many benefits **(2)**. Even today, common advice to someone who is upset or whose spirits are depressed is to tell him to concentrate his energies in his lower stomach. This in effect is a form of abdominal breathing. As one gets tired or nervous, the tension moves upward from stomach to chest until it reaches the shoulders. Conscious abdominal breathing helps check this process. It keeps one calm and in control. This same technique can be used to put oneself to sleep. Part of the technique is to think in the order exhale-inhale, rather than inhale-exhale. When walking, practice exhaling for 10 paces, and then inhale for only one pace **(3)**.

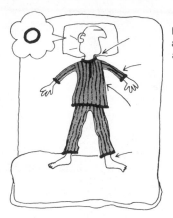

Head sideways; arms, back, and ankles relaxed

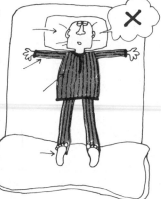

Head upward; arms straight and stiff; chest tense; feet turned up

Learn to be totally relaxed in bed

When you are ready to sleep, lie on your back with arms and legs spread slightly, close your eyes, and let all the tension flow out from your muscles.

4. Release the tension from the neck so that your head falls to the side, rather than facing straight up.

5. Release the tension from your ankles so that your feet turn outward.

6. Release the tension from your back so that it is perfectly flush with the bed. (If you have a soft bed, experiment once on the floor. A tense back will be arched enough for someone to slip a hand under, whereas a relaxed back will be flush.)

7. In this relaxed state, with eyes closed, imagine yourself sinking into the warmth of the bed. Breath slowly out-in, out-in with your stomach. If you can learn to relax like this, you will be able to sleep virtually anywhere, anytime.

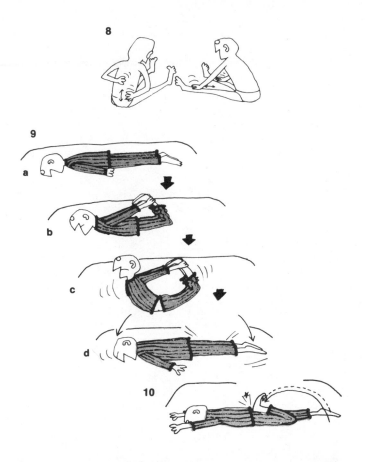

When you can't sleep

On nights when no matter how hard you try, you can't fall asleep, get up and do the following exercises:

8. Sit on the floor in just your underwear, with legs spread in front. Slowly rub each part of body with your palms from the neck down, for 5 minutes.

9. Lying face down in bed, hold ankles or toes from behind and arch back. Then release grip and, completely relaxed, let legs and shoulders fall naturally to the bed. Do this 3 times.

10. Lying face down in bed, lift legs one at a time from the knee and kick buttocks, or as far as leg will reach. Do this until it feels good.

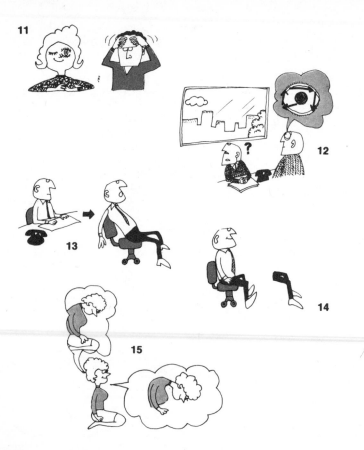

11. Beginning with fingers at forehead and thumbs at temples, massage face and head.

If you have to depend on such exercises every night in order to get to sleep, then perhaps your problems need other solutions. But the exercises are a good way to relieve the ordinary fatigue of a day at the office.

In particular, eyes can become tired without one's knowing it. At some point each day, you should rest your eyes by covering them with your hands for 30 seconds or one minute. You might also exercise them by blinking hard or by staring far out the window and moving the eyeballs up, down, and to the sides **(12).**

Another good thing to do once a day is to release all the strength from your shoulders, arms, and legs, just letting them droop lifelessly for a minute or so **(13).** One way to learn the trick of real relaxation is to tense certain muscles, for example, the muscles of your neck or toes, and then suddenly to release all tension **(14).** Notice the difference between bending your head forward and letting it fall lifelessly forward **(15).** If you can learn to do the latter, you will be one step ahead in the fight against insomnia.

Chapter 23. To Rise and Shine

Mr. Okubo, a department head in a large Japanese trading firm, spent every day either in front of his desk or in meetings, and never had any physical exercise. One summer, on vacation with his family at a mountain resort, he played golf, went bicycling and mountain climbing, and took long walks. Away from the noise and pollution of the city, breathing clean mountain air and getting plenty of sun and exercise, he began to feel like a new man.

Upon returning to his office, however, he fell back into the same busy routine, and a month later, when he tried with some confidence a physical fitness test announced in his company's weekly bulletin, he was shocked at the pitiful results.

That same test is given here. Try it, even if you think you are strong, and see how you do.

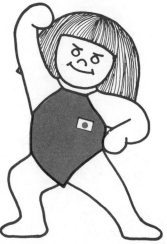

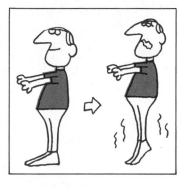

1. Balance: Raise arms in front like a diver and stand on toes with eyes closed for 20 seconds.

2. Jumping: Jump and touch knees at hip level as fast as you can 7 times.

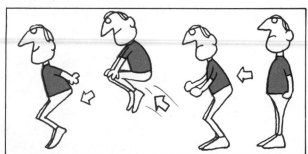

3. Sense of equilibrium: Hold left ear with left hand. Bending from the waist, touch the floor with one finger, and with that point as a center, walk in a circle 6 times in 20 seconds. Now stand and walk 10 steps straight ahead. Since you may lose your balance and fall, you should have someone stand behind for support.

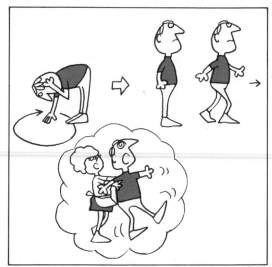

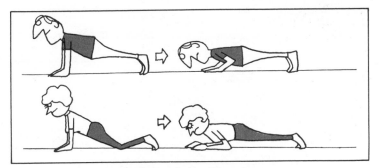

5. Strength: Do 15 push-ups.

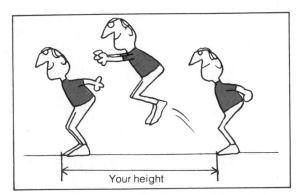

4. Leg power: From a standing position, jump a distance equivalent to your height. If you are in your twenties, jump your height plus one foot.

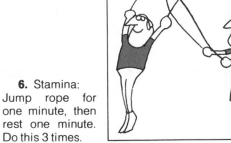

6. Stamina: Jump rope for one minute, then rest one minute. Do this 3 times.

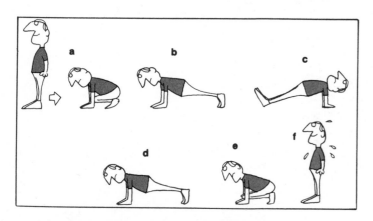

7. Agility: From a standing position, *a*) crouch and touch hands to the floor; *b*) thrust legs behind you; *c*) thrust legs in front through arms; *d*) turn over to a push-up position; *e*) return to a crouch; and *f*) finally to the original standing position. Do this series 5 times. If you are overweight, you may find step *c* difficult.

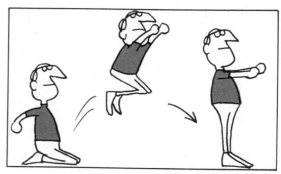

8. Agility: Jump up 5 times from a kneeling position.

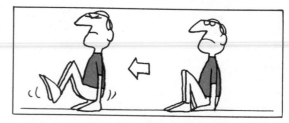

9. Dynamic balance: Sit with knees up and press yourself off the floor with hands. Hold that position for 20 seconds.

If you can do six or more of these exercises, you are in good shape. Mr. Okubo, however, was dismayed to find that he could do only four. He decided that he had better do something about this sad state of affairs, so he asked the recreation leader in his company to suggest a program of morning exercise.

Here are the exercises which the recreation leader prescribed:

10. Stretching: Raise arms in front and over head, at the same time lifting heels and rising on toes. Do this 5 times.

11. Side twisting: Sit on the floor with legs spread to shoulder width. Raise arms at sides and, keeping back straight, bend forward to touch right toe with left hand. Straighten up and repeat, touching left toe with left hand. Do this 8 times.

12. Side bends: Stand with legs apart and arms raised at sides. Without dipping knees, bend to the left and slowly return to an erect position. Repeat on the opposite side. Do this 10 times.

13. Leg thrusts: Stand erect with hands clasped behind neck. Thrust left leg as far forward as possible and push down with torso, keeping the back foot firmly planted. Return to a standing position by pushing off with left leg. Repeat with the right leg in front. Do this 10 times.

14. Sit-ups: Lie on back with knees flexed and feet flat on floor. Clasp hands behind neck and slowly sit up, touching left elbow to right knee. Return to a prone position and repeat, touching right elbow to left knee. Do this 10 times.

15. Push-ups: Be sure body is straight, with back neither sagging nor arching. Do this 10 times.

16. Compressor: Lie spread-eagled on back. Twist torso to the left, bringing right leg over and touching it to left hand. Be sure that the leg does not bend and that right arm does not leave the floor. Return slowly to the original position and repeat on the opposite side. Do this 10 times.

17. Running in place: Run in place, lifting thighs till they are parallel to the floor. Do this 15 times.

At first these exercises proved more difficult than Mr. Okubo had expected, but he did them faithfully every morning as soon as he woke up. Even on business trips abroad, he exercised in his hotel room. His facial color looked more healthy, and his sense of satisfaction and fulfillment in life increased. Soon his wife began to exercise with him. Their muscle tone, flexibility, and lung capacity improved steadily.

The lampposts lining the road to physical fitness light up one by one, just as surely as the sun comes up each morning.

Chapter 24. The Younger Man

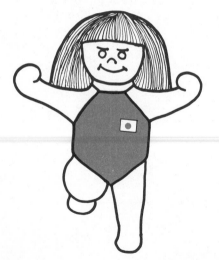

The new employees worked hard at their five-day training meeting. The schedule was rigorous and the mental strain great.

Mr. Shimada, however, was determined that nothing would prove too difficult for him. Among other things, the new employees were required to take a physical fitness test, the results of which astounded and disturbed Mr. Shimada. He had played volleyball in both high school and college and was confident in his strength, but his fitness score was much lower than he had expected. Many other employees had the lower scores of middle-aged men.

Mr. Shimada came to recognize the importance of physical fitness. As soon as he returned home, he began a modest program of exercise. Because he was renting only a small room, he couldn't do anything very active or elaborate indoors. Also, he didn't want to start a program that was too ambitious, for fear that he wouldn't be able to continue it. Therefore, he decided to try jogging.

Below is the program suggested to him by one of the recreational leaders in his company.

The 12-minute test

The aspiring jogger first assigns himself to one of five classes by measuring how far he can run in 12 minutes.

He then follows the exercise program prescribed for his level. Mr. Shimada began in the third class. The program he thus committed himself to is shown below.

Fortunately, Mr. Shimada lives near a park which is just one km (a little more than 6/10 of a mile) in circumference, so it is easy for him to estimate distances. After three weeks of training, he finally began to feel in shape. More than anything, however, he was impressed by the regular ap-pearance each morning at about 6:00 of many older joggers.

Fitness Category	Distance in 12 minutes	Oxygen Consumption
Very Poor	1 mile (1.6 km)	Under 28 ml
Poor	1-1 1/4 miles (1.6-2km)	28-34
Fair	1 1/4-1 1/2 miles (2-2.4km)	34-42
Good	1 1/2-1 3/4 miles (2.4-2.8km)	42-52
Excellent	Over 1 3/4 miles (2.8 km)	Over 52

Typical Program for Those in "Fair" Category of Fitness

Week	Distance	Walking Running	Time Goal	Frequency per week	Points per week
1	1 mile (1.6 km)	W	12'45"	5 days	10
2	1 mile	W/R	11'00"	5	15
3	1 mile	W/R	10'30"	5	15
4	1 mile	R	9'30"	5	20
5	1 mile	R	9'15"	5	20
6	1 mile	R	8'45"	3	21
	1.5 miles (2.4 km)	R	15'00"	2	
7	1 mile	R	8'30"	3	24
8	1 mile	R	7'55"	3	27
	1.5 miles	R	13'00"	2	
9	1 mile	R	7'45"	2	30
	1.5 miles	R	12'30"	2	
	2 miles (3.2 km)	R	18'00"	1	
10	1.5 miles	R	11'55"	2	31
	2 miles	R	17'00"	2	

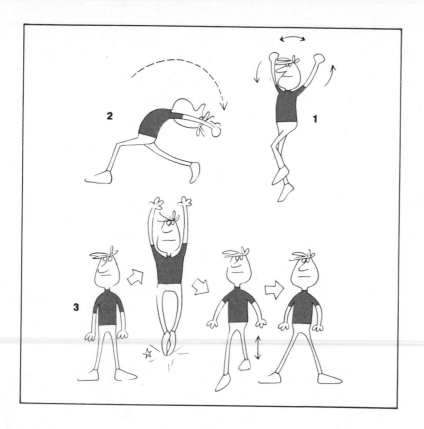

Warm-up exercises

1. Running in place: Run lightly in place while swinging arms 5 times backward and forward and 5 times up and down. Stay relaxed.

2. Back bends: Thrust one leg forward. Flexing the extended knee and bringing arms forward over head, bend backward. Repeat, extending the other leg. Do this 3 times for each leg.

3. Scissor-jumps: With upper body relaxed and legs spread slightly to the sides, jump and bring feet together. Land with legs spread, one leg forward and one back. Jump again and return to the original position. Do this for 20 seconds.

Because of the pressure of his new job, Mr. Shimada had to make a special effort to limit the number of cigarettes he smoked each day. At lunch he drank an extra carton of milk.

At the end of each day Mr. Shimada returned exhausted to his room, nostalgic for his carefree life as a student. Nevertheless, the first thing he did when he got home was a simple workout. More than anything, he considered this an exercise of his willpower.

The workout was a form of circuit training, which involves the rapid execution of a series of exercises.

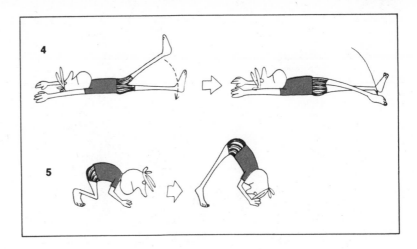

4. Leg-overs: Lie on back with arms stretched over head, palms down. Lift one leg, keeping the knee straight, slowly move it over the other leg, and touch the floor with toes. Be sure that shoulders do not leave the floor. Sitting in front of a desk all day weakens the muscles of the lower back. This exercise will strengthen those muscles. It also will help to dissipate fatigue. Do this 5 times for each leg.

5. Croquet wickets: Crouch as in the illustration, if possible with knees off the floor. Keeping elbows bent, push up with legs. Pulling in stomach and curving your back, return to the original position. Do this 8 times.

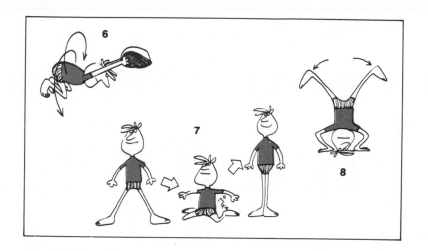

Perform the above series of exercises (4–8) in order, each the prescribed number of times, without resting. You should be able to complete the series in less than 3 minutes, but the real goal is not speed as much as the maintenance of minimum physical fitness.

Mr. Shimada himself was already quite well developed, so for him the exercises were an easy way to dissipate mental fatigue. At the same time, they build stamina, strengthen weak back and stomach muscles, and prevent stomach disorders and general stiffness.

It is no surprise that with his first month's pay, Mr. Shimada treated himself to a sweat suit and running shoes.

6. Side rolls: Kneel as in the drawing, holding a pillow in front of you. Roll over without the pillow touching the floor. Do this 5 times left and right.

7. The scrunch: Stand with legs spread wide. Sink to a squat, letting knees collapse inward, and stand again without using hands. Do this 5 times.

8. Headstand: Open and close legs 7 times while standing on head.

Chapter 25. The Office Worker

Six years after entering the employ of an electronic appliance company, two employees in their late twenties took a physical fitness test and were astounded at their low scores. Both were in the habit of playing golf once a month, and had had no sense of a decline in their general fitness since school days. The health consultant in their company, however, advised them that golf does not provide adequate exercise for young men who are interested in staying fit. He suggested that they speak with the coach of the company's volleyball team. The coach was glad to be of help, and invited them to join the team for its warm-up session.

"We always begin with running exercises," the coach said, to the dismay of the two novices. Everyone sat in a large circle on the floor facing inward, with their legs spread and their feet touching.

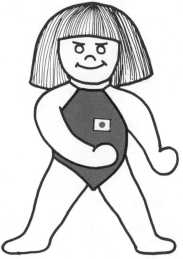

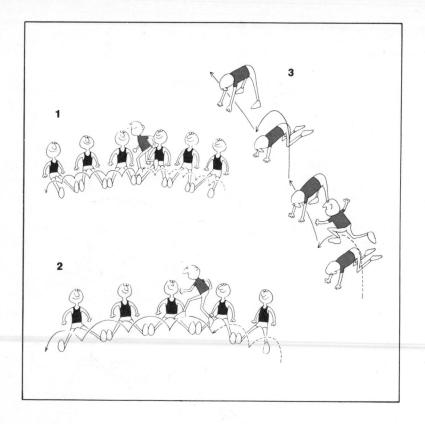

Running

If the participants are sitting in a straight line it is safe for the runner to run fast, but when they are in a circle, he may lose control if he runs too fast. He should consciously cross his outer leg over the inner slightly as he runs. Ten to twenty participants are needed for the exercise to be successful, each circling twice.

1. One by one, the participants run around the inside of the circle, stepping between the others' legs. When a runner has completed a circuit, he sits down and the next person continues.

2. The participants open their legs wider and the runner steps between the feet.

Japanese leapfrog

3. The participants increase the space between them and get down on all fours, alternately kneeling and stooping. The runner leaps over the kneelers and crawls under the stoopers.

The two novices, breathless after all the running, jumping, and crawling, were thankful for the intervals when it was their turn to rest.

Exercise with a volleyball or a basketball

Next, the coach passed out volleyballs, one to each pair of persons. Our friends the novices started batting theirs back and forth as if there were a net between them, but the coach stopped them, saying that he had other exercises in mind.

4. Catch: At 7 m (8 yards) apart, throw with the left and right hands alternately.

5. Overhead pass: Spread legs wide, and hold ball at waist. Swing down with the ball between the legs, then rise up, bend backward, and pass the ball overhead, using the whole body. The partner may move his feet to catch the ball, but he should return it in the above fashion.

6. Back-to-back pass: Do exercise 5 standing back to back. Bend backward with whole body when throwing, minimizing the wrist snap. This exercise may also be executed through the legs. Both 5 and 6 are good for weak back muscles.

7. Skier's dribble: Dribble the ball, alternating right and left hands and hopping once with each bounce like a skier, feet together and moving slowly forward. Mix large, slow hops with small faster ones.

8. Ball rolling: Bend down and roll the ball, following closely behind it. Don't go too fast or you will stumble.

9. Two-ball dribble: This is a simple basketball dribble, complicated by the use of a second ball.

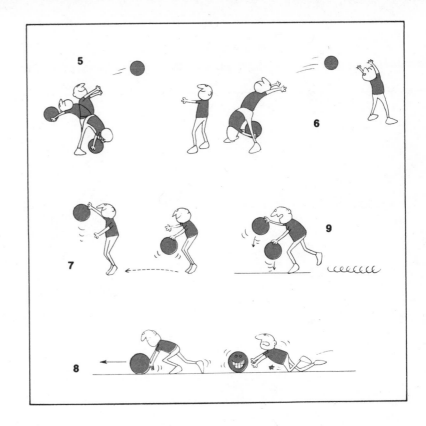

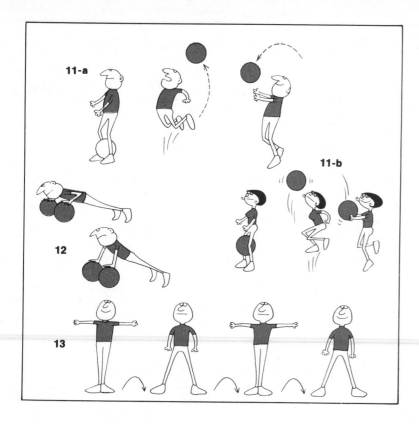

11-a

11-b

12

13

After 30 minutes of the above warm-up exercises, the coach had the two novices see if they could do the following:

10. Shoot two baskets in a row one-handed from the free-throw line.

11. Hold a basketball between the feet and jump, tossing the ball up behind and catching it in front. A simpler version of this exercise is to hold the ball between the knees, toss it up in front, and catch it.

12. Do push-ups with both hands on basketballs.

13. Do reverse jumping-jacks, spreading and closing the legs while simultaneously doing the opposite with the arms, raising them to shoulder level.

14. Bring the forehead to the floor and back while on one knee, with the arms spread for balance.

The coach said that if the two novices could do the above five tasks, they weren't totally out of shape. Unfortunately, however, one of them couldn't do 11 and 14, and the other couldn't do 12 and 14.

Women taking the same test may use a dodge ball or volleyball for 11. For the basket shooting in 10, women may use both hands and throw underhand. For 12, it is enough for women to touch their forehead to one of the balls, without pushing back up. There is no need for different requirements for men and women in 13 and

14. On the contrary, men will probably have more difficulty with 14 than women.

Cooling-down exercises

The coach came over to the somewhat embarrassed pair and suggested that they call it a day. "If you exercise too hard now, you'll be so stiff tomorrow that you won't want to continue." Then, to their surprise, he advised that they do cooling-down exercises. He led them over to a mat and had them perform the following massage exercises on each other.

One lies down and the other:

15. steps on his arches;

16. massages his Achilles tendons and calves with his feet;

17. bends his knees back and pushes;

18. massages his back and hips by climbing and kneeling on top; and

19. picks him up by the ankles and gently vibrates his legs.

As the two young men showered, they felt a sense of satisfaction that they hadn't experienced since their college days, when both had led quite vigorous lives. How long it had been since they had worked up such a healthy sweat, they couldn't remember.

As they were leaving, the coach gave them a prescription for a daily exercise routine (21–24) which they could do at home, and a check card (20). For a starter, the two vowed to stick to that routine for at least three months. They left the office building tired, but light in spirits.

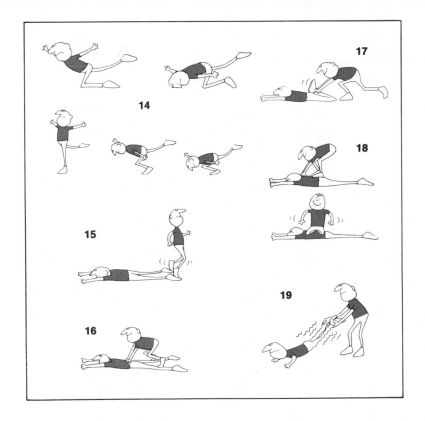

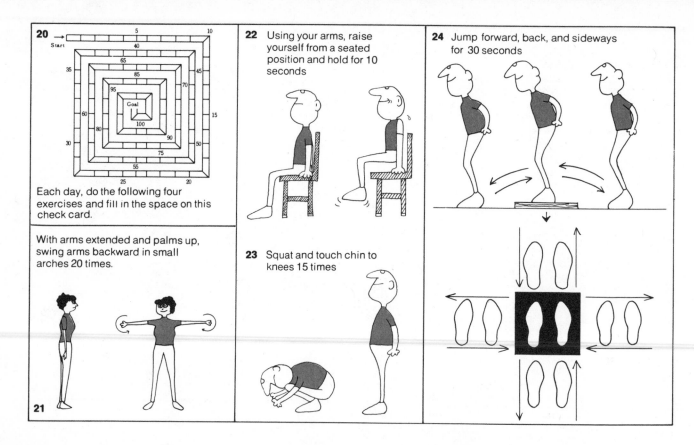

20 → Start
5 10 40 65 35 85 45 95 70 Goal 100 15 60 80 90 50 30 75 55 25 20

Each day, do the following four exercises and fill in the space on this check card.

21 With arms extended and palms up, swing arms backward in small arches 20 times.

22 Using your arms, raise yourself from a seated position and hold for 10 seconds

23 Squat and touch chin to knees 15 times

24 Jump forward, back, and sideways for 30 seconds

132

Chapter 26. The Young Businessman

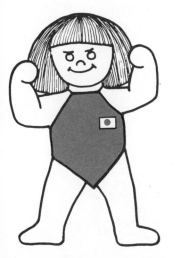

Mr. Ito is thirty-two. He lives with his wife and four-year-old daughter in company housing. His New Year's resolution was to begin and continue a physical fitness program. This decision was sparked by the poor results on the physical fitness test he took on Sports Health Day in the fall. Not only did he score in the over-forty age bracket, but he felt almost nauseous after the fourth item on the test, the zigzag dribble. It was the worried faces of his wife and colleagues as he lay on his back recovering for ten minutes which spurred him to his New Year's resolution.

He began on January 1. This is the program he set out for himself.

Become actively involved in sports

In his student days, Mr. Ito played a little tennis, but after becoming employed, he had involved himself in no other sports than an occasional swim or Ping-Pong game. And he never participated in company-sponsored events unless his attendance was required. Mr. Ito's sports plan for the year was:

January: Ski trip (two nights, three days)

Bowling class (every Saturday)

February: Ice-skating trip (one night, two days)

Bowling (Saturdays)

March: Family skiing trip (two nights, three days)

April: Tennis-club practice (once a week)

Intracompany ball-sports meet (Mr. Ito entered the tennis and Ping-Pong events)

Participate in the company bowling meet

May: Tennis practice (Wednesday and Saturday)

Class for recreation leaders

Orienteering (third Sunday)

June: Tennis practice (Wednesday and Saturday)

Orienteering (second Sunday)

July: Tennis practice (Wednesday and Sunday)

Orienteering (second Sunday)

August: Swimming (twice a week)

Rent a mountain cabin for family (three nights, four days)

Rent a beach cabin for family (one night, two days)

September: Tennis (Wednesday and Saturday)

Orienteering (third Sunday)

Badminton class (first and third Tuesdays)

October: Tennis (Saturday)

Fall athletic meet (100-m—100-yard—dash, relay race, various recreational games)

Physical fitness test

Sports sauna (twice a week)

November: Company Ping-Pong tournament

Company bowling tournament

Orienteering (first Sunday)

December: Sports sauna (twice a week)

Not only does Mr. Ito adhere faithfully to his new yearly schedule, but he also has cut down on cigarettes from forty to ten per day. Needless to say, Mrs. Ito was exceedingly happy at the changes brought about by her husband's resolution.

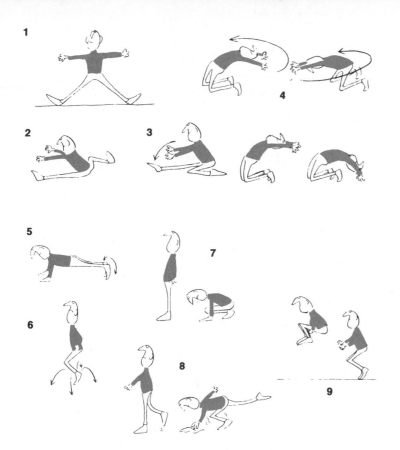

Do calisthenics daily

Morning calisthenics

Each morning before washing up, Mr. Ito chooses one or two of the following sets of exercises and spends 10 minutes doing them.

For suppleness

1. Spread legs as wide as possible. Hold for 10 seconds. From time to time, increase the width.

2. Sit in a hurdling position, alternating right and left legs forward. Do this 3 times each.

3. In a kneeling position, bend over backward and touch hands to floor behind you. Do this 3 times.

4. Kneel with knees shoulder width apart and swing arms and torso around in a large, low circle. Do this 5 times to both left and right.

For leg and back conditioning

5. Plant hands on floor in a push-up position and hop back and forth with legs together. Do this 30 seconds.

6. Hop forward, backward, and to the sides. Do this 30 seconds.

7. Stand with legs together. Bend at knees and touch palms to floor. Do this 30 times.

8. Standing on one leg with the other raised behind, bend knee and pick up a handkerchief. Do this 5 times on each leg.

9. Jump and clap hands beneath thighs. Do this 5 times.

10

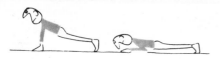

11

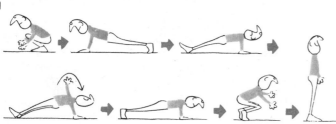

12

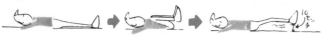

13

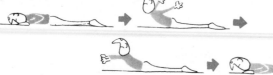

14

For strength

10. Push-ups with one hand over the other. Do this 5 times.

11. From a standing position, crouch and touch hands to floor; thrust legs behind you; thrust legs in front through arms; turn over to a push-up position; return to a crouch; and return to the original standing position. Do this 3 times.

12. Lie on back with hands clasped behind neck. Bring knees to chest and then stretch them out again, holding them 13 cm (5 inches) off floor. Do this 10 times.

13. Lie face downward and lift torso. Spread arms, extend them forward, and finally return to original position. Do this 5 times.

14. Kneel like a frog for 10 seconds.

For all-round flexibility

15. Spread legs wide and describe a large horizontal figure eight with arms and torso. Do this 10 times to both left and right.

16. Lift arms in front; swing them down and back as you raise left knee; continue arms up to behind head, swing left leg backward, and arch back; and return to starting position by simply lowering arms and leg. Do this 4 times, with both left and right leg.

17. Stand on head and open and close legs alternately to the side and in a front-back scissors. Do this 20 seconds.

During the day

As part of his commitment to daily exercise, Mr. Ito began participating vigorously in the after-lunch calisthenic sessions at his company. Also, he increased his normal walking pace by 20 percent so that he would cover 100 m (330 feet) in no more than one minute.

The three main points of Mr. Ito's physical fitness program were greater participation in sports, regular calisthenics, and walking. Anyone who begins a program like this in January and sticks to it will surely find that by spring there will be buds; by summer, flowers; and through the fall and winter, he will reap a fruitful harvest. This was certainly the case for Mr. Ito, whose reward was a great store of energy and the restoration of his youth. His example was soon followed by his wife.

Always remember the slogan: "Good health begins with physical fitness."

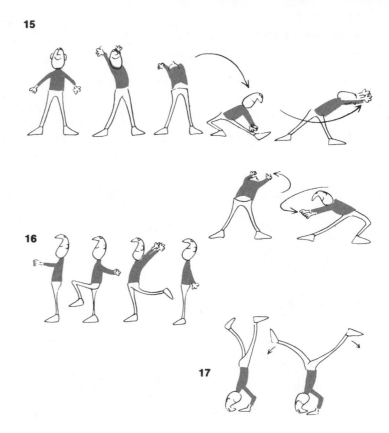

Chapter 27. The Out-of-Shape Executive

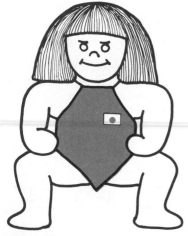

Mr. Sato, a forty-five-year-old executive, found upon taking a physical fitness test that he had the fitness of someone ten years older. Lack of exercise was the reason, and he resolved to do something about it. In the company's gym, he had watched the younger employees engaging in various sports, but he felt especially inadequate and conscious of his flabby condition when he saw one robust employee lifting weights. Hoping someday to be able to join these younger men, Mr. Sato started a program of less strenuous exercises which he could do by himself.

If you are in a similar situation, not knowing where or how to get started, try the program which was recommended to Mr. Sato.

Warm-up exercises

1. Forward backbends: From an erect position, relax upper torso and let it fall forward naturally. At first, it is all right to bend knees slightly if necessary. Gradually, try to touch fingers (and if possible, palms) to the floor. Women should try to touch wrists to the floor behind their feet. Do this 10 times.

2. Backward backbends: Spread legs and bend backward, alternately touching left heel with left hand and right heel with right hand. Do this 2 times. If you can, touch right heel with left hand, and vice versa, 2 times. Touch both heels with both hands simultaneously. Do this 2 times. Be careful not to lose balance.

3. Jumping heel touches: Rhythmically and without pause jump and touch your heels, as illustrated, 5 times.

4. Jumping toe touches: Do this exercise as illustrated 3 times. It can be done more easily with legs spread. Remember that jumping properly is more important than touching toes.

5. Touching elbows to the floor: Stand erect with hands clasped behind neck. Do a deep knee bend and, rounding the back, try to touch elbows to the floor. At first you may spread legs for this, but gradually decrease the distance between them. Do this 5 times.

6. Side slipping: In a kneeling position, shift buttocks from heels to floor at the right, then the left. Keep back straight and do not use hands for support. Do this 10 times.

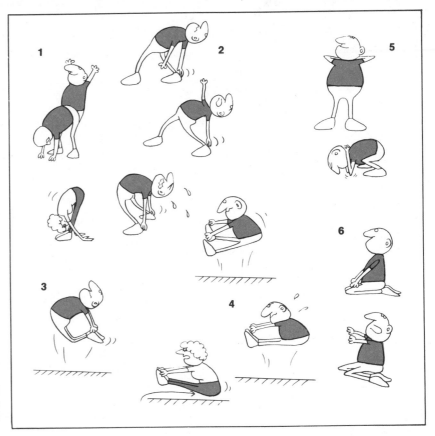

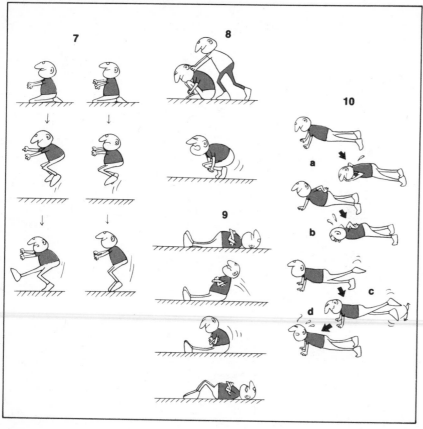

7. Jumping from a kneeling position: Jump from a kneeling position, alternately landing on right leg, left leg, and both legs. Do this 10 times.

8. Crouching stand: Sit with arms clasping knees to chest and back rounded. From that position rise to feet. If you are unable to stand have someone help by pushing your neck. Do this 3 times.

9. Sit-ups: Lie on back with arms folded across chest. Sit up slowly 3 times without lifting heels. Then lie on back with knees flexed and sit up slowly 3 times.

10. Push-ups: See if you can do the following, without regard to the number of repetitions.

a) With legs spread, touch head to the right or left hand and push back up.

b) Do a one-handed push-up, resting the other hand on back.

c) Cross and uncross legs in the air while in a push-up position.

d) Double cross and uncross legs while in a push-up position.

Exercises with a ball

Mr. Sato took 30 minutes for the above ten exercises. Then, after a 10-minute rest, he did the following exercises with a volleyball. Sometimes Mr. Sato did these exercises with a group of fellow employees, using a relay system.

Dribbling

11. While running, do basketball-type dribbles for 4 minutes.

12. While skipping, dribble, using alternating hands, for 4 minutes.

13. Two-quarter time dribble; 3/4 time dribble as in 11 for 4 minutes.

14. Spin alternately to the left and right while dribbling for 4 minutes.

15. Rest for 5 minutes.

16. If you have time, repeat exercises 11 to 13 above, using two balls.

17. Rest for another 5 minutes.

18. Make one circuit dribbling ball on thighs. Do not use hands, and do not let ball touch knees or it will bound away from you.

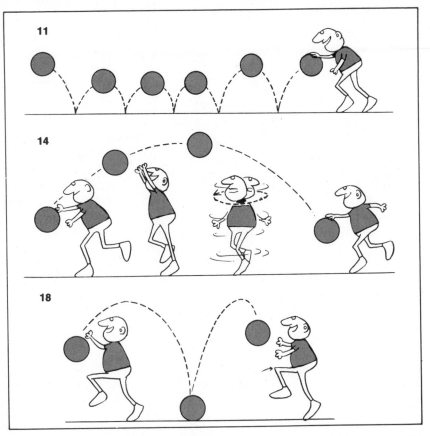

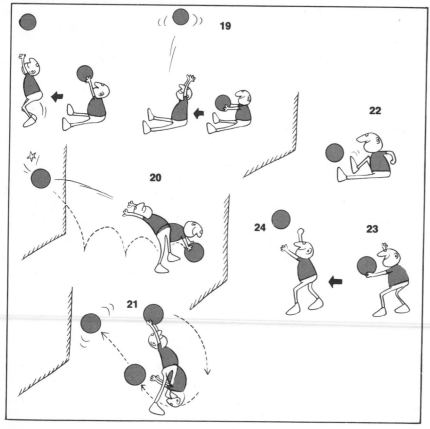

Passing

19. Catch: Toss the ball into the air and catch it while sitting on the floor with legs spread. Also try tossing it up and then standing to catch it.

20. Back pass over the head: Throw the ball over your head against the wall of the gym and retrieve it from between legs.

21. Back pass between the legs: Throw the ball between legs as high as possible.

22. From a sitting position, kick the ball against the wall.

23. Spike the ball as you would a volleyball so that it hits the floor once before rebounding off the wall.

24. Serve the ball overhead as in volleyball, directly against the wall.

At the end of his first workout, Mr. Sato was tired and sweaty but in high spirits. He slowly ran several laps and went through the regular cooling-down exercises before heading for the shower.

Chapter 28. The Fit Executive

Three months after embarking on his new fitness program, Mr. Sato had become a regular at his company's gymnasium, with at least one vigorous workout per week. He had lost his flab, his muscle tone was good, and his spirits at home and at the office were high.

Let us now look at the updated version of his exercise program.

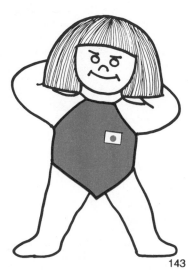

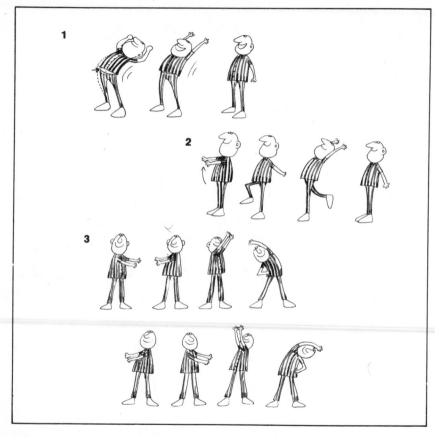

Morning

1. Lung expansions: As soon as he wakes, Mr. Sato opens the window and takes 16 deep breaths.

2. Arm, leg, and back stretching: This exercise is to be done rhythmically in quarter time. Start by standing straight with arms at side; raise arms in front to shoulder height on first beat; on second beat, swing arms back and raise one knee; on the third beat swing arms forward and up and leg back, bending the body back; rest on the fourth beat.

3. Side stretching: As illustrated, swing arms and stretch side muscles in quarter time.

4. Body rub: In underpants only, massage whole body beginning with legs and thighs and continuing to arms, belly, chest, neck, and face. Rub for about 5 minutes, until each part is warmed. Mr. Sato gives particular attention to his belly because of the stomach disorders which used to bother him.

5. When the weather is good, he swings a golf club or a tennis racket in the yard. Thirty strokes with a club, bat, or racket not only is good exercise but also keeps one in proper form for a favorite sport.

Noon

At noon, Mr. Sato often joins the younger employees for basketball. Sometimes, however, he works at the "ten-part fitness test" (6–15) introduced to him by one of the recreation leaders.

6. With arms raised in front like a diver, close eyes and balance on toes for 30 seconds.

7. Jump and touch knees at hip level 10 times in quick succession.

8. Touch one finger to the floor and, with that point as a center, walk around 6 times in 20 seconds. Straighten up and walk 10 steps forward. If you have not been doing any exercises which involve spinning, you may lose your balance and fall. If so, reduce the number of revolutions.

9. Do a backward standing broad jump more than two-thirds your height.

10. Do 15 push-ups.

11. Jump rope for one minute and rest one minute 3 times.

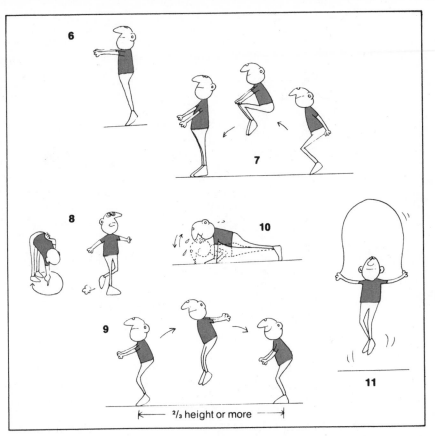

²/₃ height or more

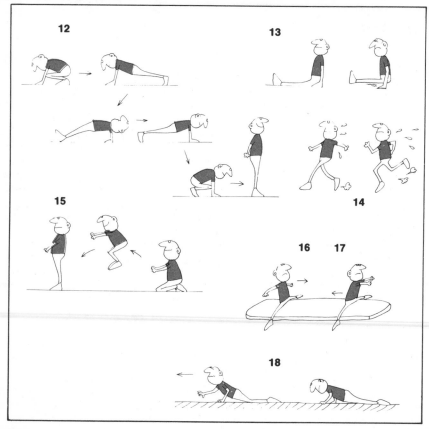

12. From a standing position, *a*) crouch and touch hands to the floor; *b*) thrust legs behind you; *c*) thrust legs in front through arms; *d*) turn over to a push-up position; *e*) return to a crouch; and then *f*) to a standing position. Do this 7 times.

13. Sit on the floor with legs extended together. Press yourself off the floor with hands and hold for 10 seconds.

14. Walk and run one km (0.6 mile) in 4 minutes.

15. Jump from a kneeling to a standing position 10 times in succession.

Of the ten tasks, there were still four that Mr. Sato could not do. The accomplishment of all ten was his next goal. Women may cut the number of repetitions in half and aim to execute at least seven of the ten.

Evening

Mr. Sato often begins his evening workout on a long mat.

16. Quickly walk the length of the mat with feet straddling it.

17. Repeat backward, keeping an erect posture.

18. Pull yourself forward on stomach from one end of mat to the other using arms only.

19. Hop the length of the mat in zigzag fashion with legs together.

20. Repeat the zigzaging hop with a ball, dribbling once with each hop.

21. Do a rhythmic series of rabbit hops: jump, kneel, breathe; jump, kneel, breathe.

22. Do a slow forward somersault, crossing legs in the process, and stand up facing in the opposite direction. Continue with a backward somersault, crossing legs again, and stand up facing in the original direction.

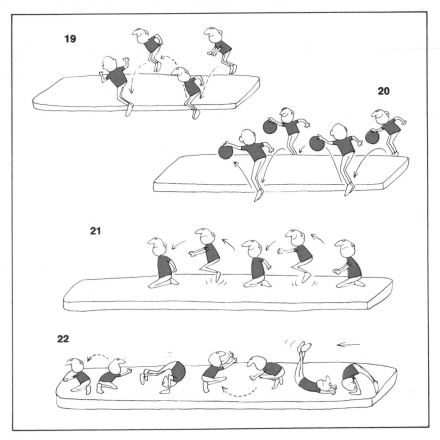

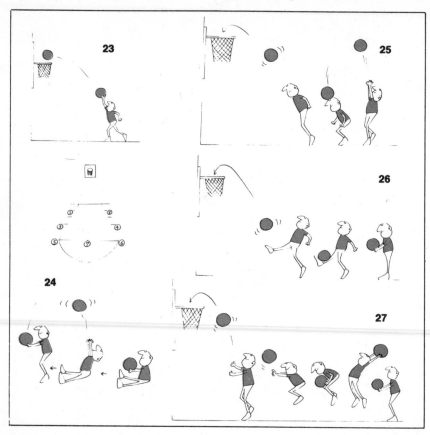

23. After finishing with the mat, Mr. Sato shot baskets, beginning at the spot marked "1" in the diagram. When he had made a basket, he would move to spot number 2 and then the other spots in order, finally shooting 2 single-handed baskets in a row from the free-throw line. It was his rule not to move from one spot to the next until he had made a basket, and that he not finish until he had thrown 2 free throws in a row.

Basket shooting of this kind is a good cooling-down exercise. It also can be a good group game.

Since Mr. Sato had a meeting with friends and time was short, he finished his workout with the following exercises using a volleyball:

24. Sit on the floor, toss the ball into the air, and jump to catch it. Do this 3 times.

25. Throw the ball into the air and try to "head" it into a basket. Do this 5 times.

26. Drop-kick the ball into the basket from the free-throw line. Take 5 tries.

27. Jump as if to do an overhead jump shot, but instead bring the ball down for an underhand shot. The ball must leave your hands before your feet reach the floor. Do this 3 times.

After showering, Mr. Sato went off to his meeting fit and refreshed. His friends all commented on how young and healthy he looked.

Chapter 29. Calisthenics with a Partner

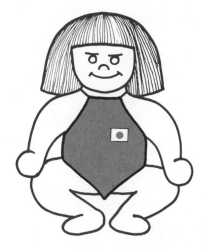

Company health management programs have placed increasing emphasis on the importance of physical fitness among employees. The most common and effective measure has been the introduction of group calisthenics before work in the morning, during the lunch hour, or perhaps during a break in the afternoon. In addition to the maintenance of physical fitness, the morning calisthenics help gather scattered thoughts into a collective will. In the afternoon, calisthenics can provide a needed change of pace or relief from tension.

Participants in most calisthenic sessions in Japan face in the same direction and perform the various exercises separated from one another. Calisthenics may basically be an individual matter, but such uniformity and isolation tend to negate the inherent interest potential of exercising. The harder and longer one works at any given exercise, the more likely it is that the activity will become puppetlike and mechanical. To be effective, a calisthenic program should be diverse and always changing.

I would like in this chapter to introduce a program which was designed for exercise in pairs. This program was adopted some time ago by certain Japanese companies and has proved very successful, especially in creating healthy relations between superiors and subordinates in a strongly vertical society. Each day partners change, so that department heads work out with secretaries, and supervisors with new employees. Not only does the working environment improve, but calisthenics become attractive rather than neglected. Absenteeism also has declined noticeably. Musical accompaniment contributes to the program's popularity.

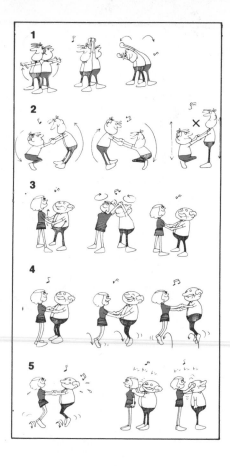

1. Side bends: Stand back to back and slowly raise arms in front and overhead. Join hands with partner and slowly bend to the sides.

2. Seesaw: Face and hold hands. Seesaw up and down, with one partner squatting while the other stands, and vice versa. At first there will be a tendency to move straight up and down like pistons, but with practice, the partners will learn a kind of rocking motion that describes the arcs of parentheses. This is good conditioning for the legs and back.

3. Overhead twirl: Face and hold hands. Swing arms to the left, to the right, and then back to the left; take one step and swing arms overhead and turn back to back. Continue swing of arms and turn until you've come all the way around. If this is difficult, you may release the outer hand as you turn. If there is space, step back and forth as you swing arms. This exercise will help keep a trim waistline.

4. Hopping: Face and hold hands. With feet together, make one big jump to the left and one to the right, followed by 3 smaller left-right-left jumps. The rhythm of this is *one*, rest; *two*, rest; *one, two, three,* rest.

5. Shoulder massage: To a count of 16 beats, take turns pounding each other's shoulders.

The exercises themselves may not seem like much, but when done in pairs they can be very effective. Here are some more suggestions.

6. Foot wrestling: Hold hands and try to step on each other's feet. The first to do this twice wins. This is good for agility and endurance.

7. Back lifts: Standing back to back, hold partner's wrists and lift him onto your back. Bear most of his weight with your shoulders or he will be uncomfortable. Once his feet have left the floor, turn slowly in a circle. Then trade positions. The person being lifted should relax and take care not to lift his knees up, or both will fall over.

8. Side bends: This is more effective done with a partner than alone. Stand back to back with legs apart and arms tightly locked and bend from side to side.

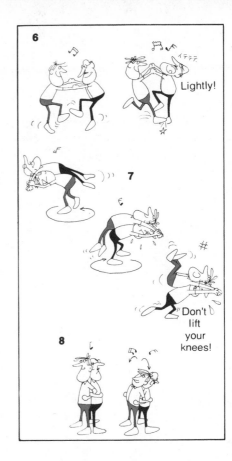

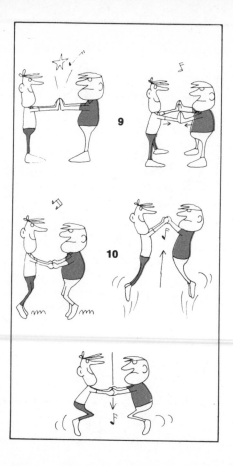

9. Palm pushing: Stand face to face with arms stretched in front. Push palms together lightly for 3 counts. On the fourth count, spread arms and give a stronger push. Use forearms rather than shoulders to push.

10. Jump and squat: Standing face to face and with hands together jump lightly for 3 counts and squatting on the fourth. If both partners are young, they may jump high on the third count and land squatting on the fourth. This exercise strengthens legs and back.

11. Arm wrestling: Stand face to face with right arms locked, left hands on hips, and feet together. Try to make partner lose his balance.

12. Scissors, paper, and stone: Stand facing one yard apart. Jump lightly for 2 counts. On the third count land with legs open to the side (scissors), open to the front and back (paper), or together (stone). If you both land in the same position, begin again. Scissors cut paper, paper wraps stone, and stone crushes scissors.

Choose games, exercises, and music which will suit the conditions and atmosphere of your company or factory. For variety, introduce new ideas on occasion.

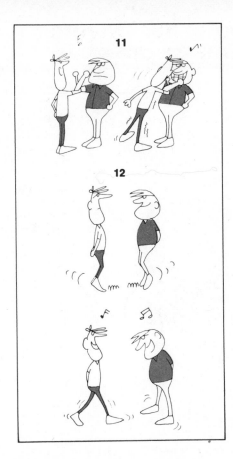

Chapter 30. Drivers

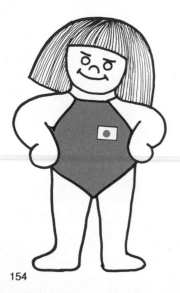

Mr. Furuta is a conscientious taxi driver who is proud of his perfect driving record and trusted by his customers. Needless to say, the business of navigating the sometimes fierce traffic conditions of a large city can be a strain on the nerves. It is doubly important, therefore, that a driver never become riled or irritable. Mr. Furuta is thankful for his wife's cheerfulness each morning as she sees him off to work. But his hours are long and irregular, and recently he began to suffer from stomach disorders and general fatigue. He tried vitamins and other drugs, but to no avail. Finally, he started a physical fitness program.

After only one month, Mr. Furuta's condition improved so markedly that he actively began to encourage his fellow cab drivers to follow his example. Let us look at a day in the life of the new Mr. Furuta.

At 6:00 in the morning, he rises and does a series of exercises of his own choice, each repeated 3 times.

1. Kneel with hands clasped behind neck, and pull elbows back as far as possible.

2. Clasp hands behind lower back with palms down, and stretch arms.

3. Rotate neck to the front, back, and sides.

4. Touch toes in a sitting position with legs stretched out.

5. Kneel, sitting on heels, with arms stretched overhead, and bend backward to the floor.

6. Lie on back and touch toes to the floor above head.

7. Stand erect with hands on hips and stretch the legs as far as possible to the sides.

8. From a standing position, raise the arms in front and at the same time do a deep knee bend without letting the heels leave the floor.

When he has finished, Mr. Furuta dresses and takes a 10-minute spin on his bicycle. Not only taxi drivers but anyone who spends time at the wheel lacks leg exercise. Since old age is said to begin in the legs, Mr. Furuta is wise to delay that process by riding his bicycle, even if for only 10 minutes a day. On rainy days, he does 20 deep knee bends instead of riding the bike.

The morning workout takes about 30 minutes. Then he washes, reads the paper, and at 7:00 eats a hearty breakfast of ham, eggs, milk, and fruit.

At 8:00 he leaves in his cab for two regular pickups and then continues work until about 12:30. Sometimes during the morning, when he lets a passenger out and there is no other fare waiting, he parks the cab (if he can find a space) and does some quick exercises.

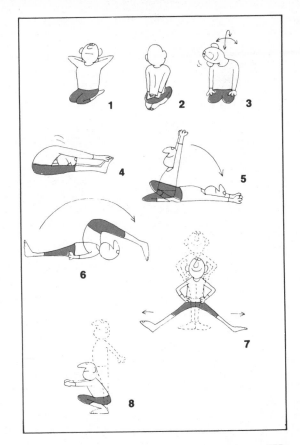

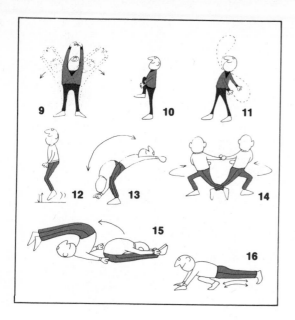

9. Stretch trunk to the sides, with hands clasped high over the head.

10. Standing erect clasp one knee at a time to the chest.

11. With a slight bounce in the knees, describe figure eights in the air with arms.

Mr. Furuta takes only 30 seconds for these exercises, and does them 3 to 5 times each day.

He takes an hour for lunch with other taxi drivers at about 12:30, and after a short nap in his car and a quick 30 seconds of exercises, he heads back into the traffic.

Toward evening, after a long, hard day, Mr. Furuta heads for the dispatcher to turn in his earnings. About once a week, after work, he stops off at a sports sauna near the garage before returning home. He starts there with a series of warm-ups:

12. Jumping (20 or 30 times)

13. Backbends (5–10)

14. Side twisting (5–10)

15. Prone backbends (5–10)

16. Leg stretching (10–20)

At the sports sauna there is a variety of courses to choose from —the general course, the stamina course, the body-building course, and others, each divided into five levels. Mr. Furuta was advised to begin at the third level of the general course, which is shown below.

One day, as Mr. Furuta was about to take a sauna after his workout, he was approached by one of the trainers, who suggested that Mr. Furuta was ready to advance to the fourth level of the general course. That advice, plus the sauna, put Mr. Furuta in a good mood as he headed back to his taxi at about 7:00.

Mr. Furuta entered the traffic again, intending to return straight home, but was hailed almost immediately by a customer. The proposed trip would take him more than an hour out of his way, but since he was in good spirits, Mr. Furuta undertook the job. Fortunately, traffic was light and the trip easy. Home by 8:30, he sat down to a half-pint of sake, a big meal of fish, meat, and vegetables, and an enjoyable evening with his family.

Because he had already worked out at the sauna, he skipped his usual pre-bath exercises, but ordinarily before taking a bath, Mr. Furuta would do the following:

	Level 1	Level 2	Level 3	Level 4	Level 5
Bar Press (**17**)	——	——	10 times (3 strands)	10 times (4 strands)	10 times (5 strands)
Cycling (30 km/hour or18 mph) (**18**)	2 minutes	3 minutes	3 minutes	4 minutes	5 minutes
Rowing (**19**)	20 strokes	30 strokes	50 strokes	70 strokes	100 strokes
Basket Throwing (**20**)	10 throws	15 throws	20 throws	25 throws	30 throws
Horse Vaulting (**21**)	5 times	7 times	10 times	15 times	20 times
Fencing Strokes (**22**)	——	20 strokes	30 strokes	40 strokes	50 strokes
Rack Climbing (**23**)	5 times	5 times	7 times	10 times	10 times
Jumping 20 cm or 8 inches (**24**)	——	10 times	20 times	25 times	30 times
Place Running (**25**)	500 paces (3 minutes)	500 paces (3 minutes)	700 paces (4 minutes)	800 paces (5 minutes)	1,000 paces (6 minutes)

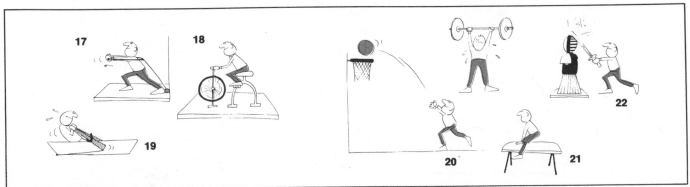

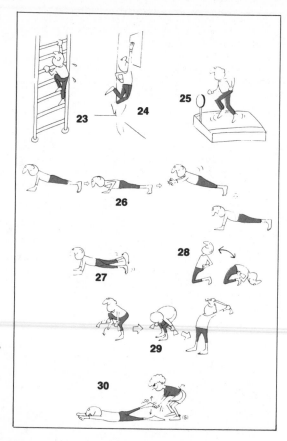

26. Five hand-clap push-ups.

27. Push-up position side-jumps with arms stationary.

28. Kneeling backbends: Kneeling in an upright position, with hands supporting the lower back, bend over backward and touch head to the floor. Do this 2 times.

29. Hold a towel taut with both hands at shoulder width. Bend forward at the waist, step over the towel one foot at a time, and bring the towel behind the back and over the head. Do this 3 times.

30. Lie face down and have someone gently shake your legs one by one.

By the time Mr. Furuta has finished his bath, it is usually 10:30, bedtime for an early riser. Given his occupation, one cannot but be impressed by the amount of exercise Mr. Furuta fits into his busy and unpredictable schedule. The more one drives, the more necessary it is to find ways to make simple exercise a part of the daily routine.

Chapter 31. A Physical Fitness Test

PART IV. PROGRAMS FOR WOMEN

The tests in this chapter are meant for women or for children under fourteen. Points gained in each test can be added up for total score.

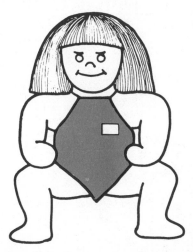

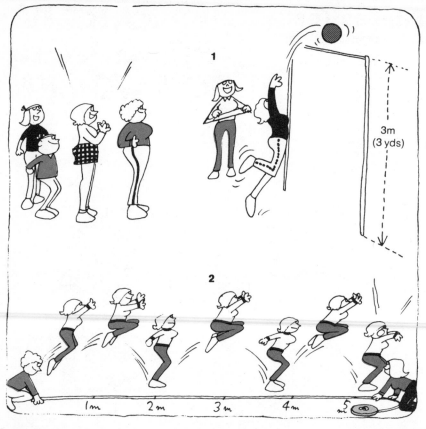

1. Basketball throw: Fix a string or rope horizontally 3 m (3 yards) above the ground. How many times can you toss a ball over the string in 30 seconds?

10 times = 1 point
13 times = 2 points
16 times = 3 points
19 times = 4 points
22 times = 5 points

2. Continuous standing broad jumps: From a standing start, how far can you move in 3 jumps with feet together?

3.5 m (11 feet) = 1 point
4.25 m (14 feet) = 2 points
5.0 m (16 feet) = 3 points
5.75 m (19 feet) = 4 points
6.50 m (21 feet) = 5 points

3m
(3 yds)

1m   2m   3m   4m   5

3. Medicine-ball throw: How far can you move a 2-kg (4.4-pound) medicine ball in 3 successive throws either overhand or underhand?

15 m (49 feet) = 1 point
18 m (59 feet) = 2 points
21 m (69 feet) = 3 points
24 m (79 feet) = 4 points
27 m (89 feet) = 5 points

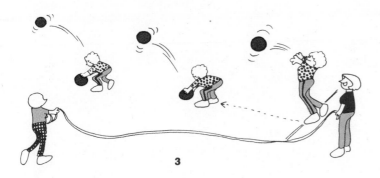

3

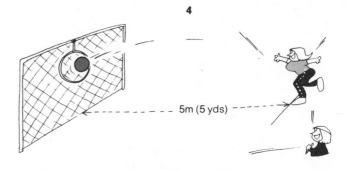

4

5m (5 yds)

4. Hoop ball: Hang a hoop at about the height of a soccer goal. From 5 m away, how many times out of 5 can you throw an 800-gram (28-ounce) exercise ball through the hoop? You get 1 point for each hoop.

5. Horizontal bar vaulting: How many times in 30 seconds can you vault over a bar set 60 cm (2 feet) above the ground?

10 times = 1 point
15 times = 2 points
20 times = 3 points
25 times = 4 points
30 times = 5 points

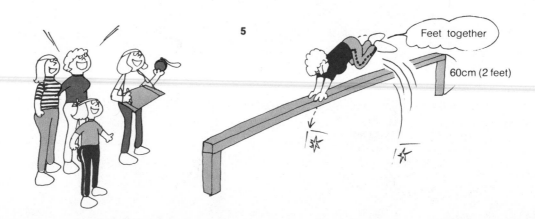

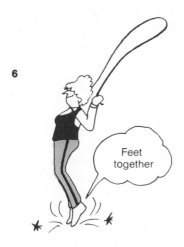

6

Feet together

6. Jumping rope: How many times can you jump rope in 30 seconds?

25 times = 1 point
30 times = 2 points
35 times = 3 points
40 times = 4 points
45 times = 5 points

7. Diagonal chin-ups: Lean back from a 1 m, 20 cm (4 feet) high horizontal bar so that your arms are at a right angle to your body. How many chin-ups can you do in that position in 30 seconds? (Chin must go above bar for one time.)

5 times = 1 point
10 times = 2 points
15 times = 3 points
20 times = 4 points
25 times = 5 points

7

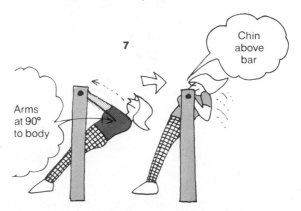

Chin above bar

Arms at 90° to body

8. A 400-m (440-yard) run: How fast can you run this distance?

    2'45" = 1 point
    2'30" = 2 points
    2'15" = 3 points
    2'00" = 4 points
    1'45" = 5 points

9. A 4-km (2.4-mile) walk: If you can walk this distance without resting, regardless of how long it takes, you get 5 points.

A perfect score for the nine tests is 45 points. How did you do?

Let this be an incentive to take up a sport or a physical fitness program.

8

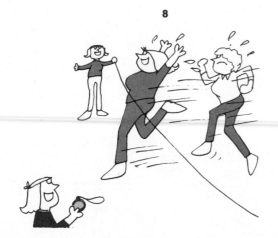

9

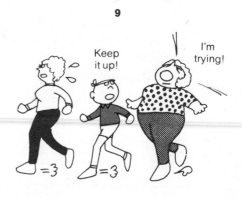

Chapter 32. Younger Women

While the attraction to natural and physical beauty is universal, women more than men actively strive to make themselves beautiful. Young women in particular take great pains in the choice of clothes and accessories, in the care of their skin, and in the use of cosmetics. Unfortunately, however, this care does not always extend to physical fitness or to beauty in movement. And whenever bothered by stiff shoulders, aching legs, headaches, or insomnia, many women rely on drugs, or simply bear up as best they can.

Neither idle wishing nor chemicals will slow the passing of youth, which really is only a dream anyhow. Sooner or later, reality forces itself upon us. Physical fitness, therefore, is not a measure of vanity. It is rather a measure toward health, a way to lead a life free from the regrets and ills which come with middle age.

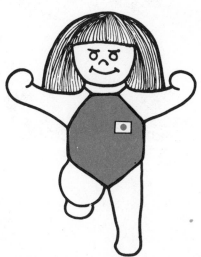

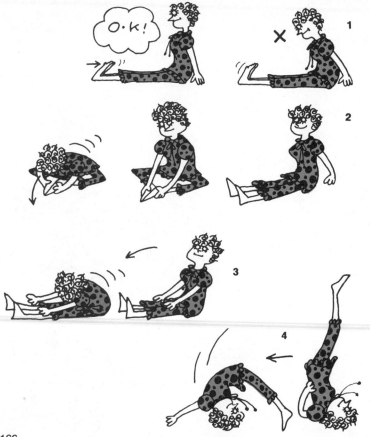

Secret exercises for beauty

The following four exercises have been adopted from yoga for their beauty and health benefits. Do them for 2 minutes after a shower or a bath, or just before going to bed. They are especially good if you have trouble sleeping.

1. Sit on the floor with legs stretched straight out. Keeping back straight, pull toes back toward knees and push heels forward. This looks like an exercise for the ankles, but it really is meant for the waistline.

2. Still seated, hold the bottoms of your feet together with hands, pull them as close to you as possible, and bend forward from the waist. Try to bring face all the way to floor, though this will be difficult at first. Consider this stiffness a loss of youth which can be brought back over time with patience and persistence. These first two exercises should be considered a pair.

3. Sit with legs stretched out in front, and bend forward from waist.

4. Lie flat on back, bring legs and torso up, and touch floor behind head with toes.

With these four exercises alone, you can improve your health and beauty. They will stimulate your spinal column, freeing up blockages of the autonomous nervous system, and let you tap more directly the great forces of life which are within you.

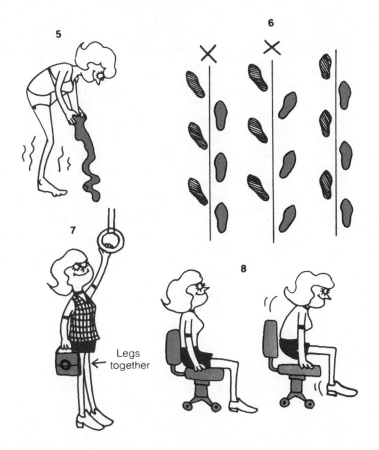

Tips for staying young

5. When putting on and taking off footwear, stand on one leg rather than sitting down.

6. When walking or running, point feet straight ahead.

7. When standing on a train or bus, keep balance by holding thighs tightly together.

8. If you work at a desk, raise yourself from your seat with arms and hold for 3 seconds twice a day.

Legs ← together

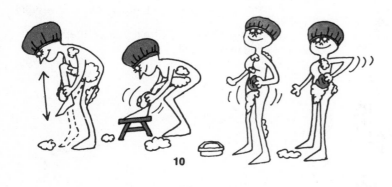

10

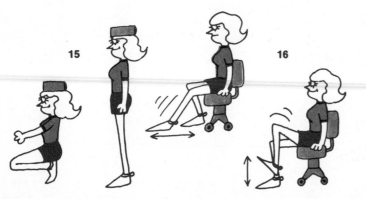

15

16

9. Rinse eyes for a bright, cool look. If they are tired, open them wide and shut them tight alternately, and then massage them lightly with fingertips.

10. When showering (or bathing, as in the illustration, in a Japanese-style bath), move your leg, stomach, or whatever part of the body you are washing, instead of moving the hand holding the washcloth.

11. Once a day, rest hand on abdomen and tense the stomach muscles so hard that you begin to quiver and hold for 6 seconds.

12. Use the staircase for up to three flights as if there were no elevator in the building.

13. Try your hand (or legs) at sports that you've never played before.

14. When walking, exhale slowly only once over the course of each 10 paces.

With only a minimum of effort you should be able to adopt these ten habits into your daily life. It is a matter of will, pure and simple, a matter either of holding on to youth or of letting it go.

A simple daily exercise program

Fix a place in your daily routine for the following five exercises. Do them faithfully, and you will find a marked improvement in your condition within a month.

15. Do 5 deep knee bends with a book balanced on head.

16. In a seated position, lift legs one at a time; also extend them front and back. Do this 3 times for each leg.

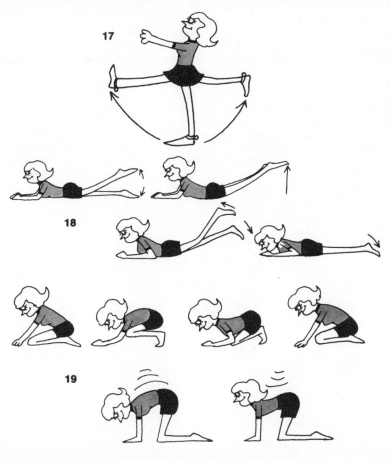

17. Stand on one leg and swing the other back and forth in a large arc. Do this 5 times for each leg.

18. Lying on your stomach, lift one leg, then lift the other to join it. Spread and close the legs, and lower them. Do this 3 times.

19. Kneel, sitting on heels, with hands on the floor in front. Bend forward with back bowed inward. Round back and return to original position. Do this 5 times. If it is difficult, try it on all fours, alternately relaxing stomach with a bowed back, and tensing stomach with a rounded back.

A well-exercised body feels more fully the rewards of being alive. And this is totally different from the satisfaction of losing weight. Exercise is a fundamental life discipline. It can bring health and youthfulness, and if it is securely integrated into one's daily life and awareness it can be an ever-renewable source of joy. It is the privilege of the cultivated woman to be immersed in this special sense of joy. The happiness of full womanhood is within your reach, within the fitness of body that lies behind fitness of mind and soul.

Chapter 33. Shopping

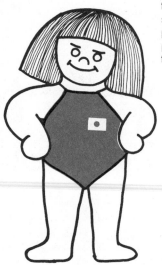

Many Japanese housewives shop almost every day, usually at nearby shops, for the day's food. Occasionally, though, they go to the more distant department stores, which in Japan also sell food products, traveling by taxi or public transportation. Such excursions, both near and far, can be a valuable source of exercise for the otherwise housebound woman, and should be recognized as such. It is unfortunate that some women are too easily tempted by the luxury of ordering by phone and having the merchandise delivered. In this chapter, I will discuss ways in which the exercise potential of the shopping excursion can be maximized.

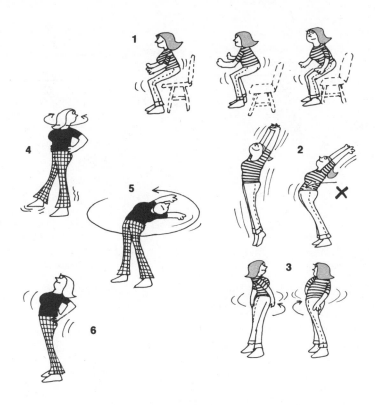

Before shopping

Almost every woman getting ready for a shopping excursion will take a moment to dress properly, put her hair in order, and check to make sure she has her purse and shopping bag. How about adding the following three quickie exercises to your regular preparations?

1. Half-sitting: Begin the motion to sit, but stop just before reaching the edge of the chair. Stand up again and do the same to the right of the chair, then to the left.

2. Stretching: Intertwine fingers and, on tiptoe, stretch arms high above head, palms facing the ceiling. Keep back straight and do not let stomach protrude.

3. Torso twisting: Hold arms loosely at your sides and twist torso to the left and right.

These three exercises can be done in just 10 seconds, but if they are done five times a day, 365 days a year, that is not an insignificant amount of exercise and will make a noticeable difference in appearance and fitness.

Before going out in the afternoon, do the following set of exercises.

4. Balancing on one leg with hands on hips or raised at the side, slowly turn neck from side to side. Difficulty in keeping balance is a sign of aging.

5. Torso swinging: With legs spread to shoulder width, swing torso and arms in large circles, first to left, then to right.

6. Back arching: Press muscles which border lower backbone with thumbs as in *shiatsu* (Japanese pressure-point massage), and arch back.

171

Advice for the neighborhood shopping trip

7. The farther and faster you walk, the more calories you use.

8. Carry purchases home yourself, rather than having them delivered. Unused muscles tend to atrophy.

9. If you are carrying something in one hand, occasionally change it to the other. Also, hold a shopping bag with only one or two fingers.

10. There is no reason to walk slowly when you are carrying a shopping bag. Walk briskly, even if you are carrying something heavy.

11. Walk with an erect posture. There is nothing more unsightly than slouching home with shopping bags in hand.

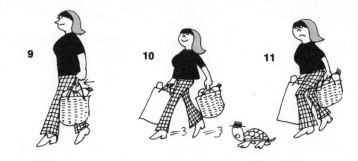

In the department store

12. If you are going to the third or fourth floors, use the staircase rather than the elevator.

13. When coming back down, assume that there is no elevator or escalator.

14. On occasions when you do use the escalator, balance on one foot.

15. When you sit down for a short rest, massage shoulders, arms, and legs.

16. If you are taking home a heavy load, divide it evenly in two bags rather than carrying it one-handed.

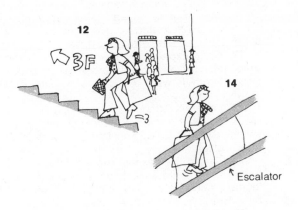

Escalator

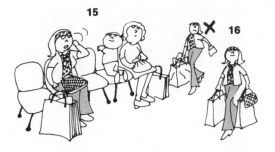

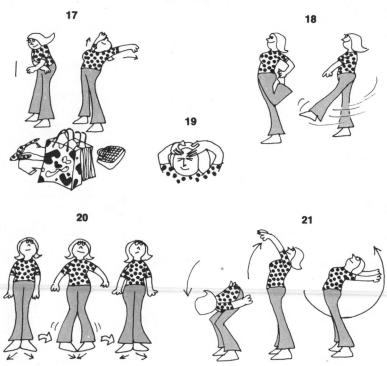

17

18

19

20

21

After shopping

After a long shopping expedition, one is understandably tired, and perhaps suffering from a headache because of the crowds in the department store. To relieve tension and fatigue, turn on the radio or stereo and do the following exercises.

17. Chest expansion and embracing: Spread arms diagonally up and back, and expand chest; then bend slightly forward and embrace yourself. Repeat slowly 3 times.

18. Leg relaxation: Stand on one leg. Lift and press the other against the back of thigh, then let it swing naturally down and forward. Do this 2 times right and left.

19. *Shiatsu* (finger massage) for the head: Place palms on the sides of head and press hard with thumbs, concentrating on the places where it feels best. This is good for a headache.

20. Duck-toes, pigeon-toes: Stand at attention with feet opened about 60°. Move sideways by turning toes alternately inward, then outward. This is a way to revive one's spirits.

21. Forward-bending, back-arching arm swings: Swing arms forward and down, and bend at waist and knees. Then rise up at knees and waist, lifting arms up, and arch back.

Chapter 34. At Home

Mrs. Ashizawa is thirty-five and has two children, a daughter in the eighth grade and a son in the fifth. Her husband is thirty-six and works in a large business firm. They live in a small apartment on the second floor of a large apartment complex. Mrs. Ashizawa is 5'3", and before starting her physical fitness program, she weighed 132 pounds.

One weekend, she participated with the rest of her family in an athletic day at her husband's company. In one corner of the gymnasium, physical fitness tests were being administered. Since she had been quite athletic in high school, Mrs. Ashizawa submitted herself to a test while her family cheered her on. She scored 12 points on the repetition side jump, 11 on the vertical jump, 8 on the hand grip, 16 on the zigzag dribble, and 7 on speed walking for a total of 54 points. This was a disappointment for Mrs. Ashizawa, since 54 points placed her in the thirty-five to thirty-nine age bracket. The diagnosis of the physical fitness consultant was that Mrs. Ashizawa's weight, 25 pounds heavier than when she married, was excessive, and that her stamina was low. Mrs. Ashizawa was stunned by the decline in her physical condition and resolved to take the consultant's advice for a regular exercise program.

Two months and 5 pounds later, she looked trimmer and felt more energetic than ever. She was particularly pleased when her children and husband commented on how good she looked. Free now from the heaviest duties of child rearing, she does embroidery, takes flower-arranging lessons, and is active in a ballet class for mothers.

Let us look at the exercise program which brought so much happiness to Mrs. Ashizawa.

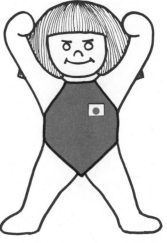

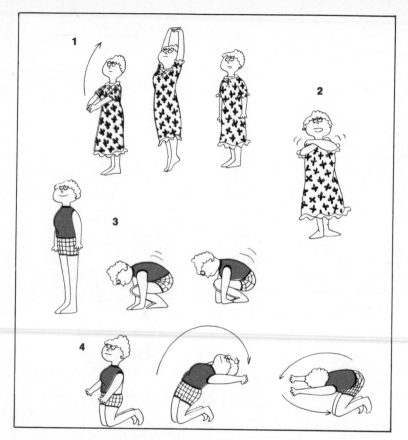

Indoor exercises

First thing every morning

1. Lace fingers together and raise arms high over head, palms toward the ceiling, as you rise to toes and stretch. Relax and let arms fall naturally to sides. Do this twice.

2. Massage shoulders for one minute.

Calisthenics (3 times a week)

3. Stand with feet together. Bend deeply at the knees, keeping heels in place, and touch palms to the floor. Do this 10 times.

4. Kneel and swing arms and torso in a large, low circle 5 times to both right and left.

5. Sit with legs stretched in front and arms folded. You may bend knees slightly if necessary. Raise feet from the floor and swing 180° without losing balance. Let feet down briefly and then swing back to the original position. If this is difficult with arms folded, you may leave them free. However, you must not touch the floor with hands.

6. Sit on the floor with knees up and hands holding ankles tightly. From that position, curl your back and come to feet without releasing hands, and then roll over backward. Try to return to the original position without using the reverse momentum of the back roll. This may seem easy, but it is surprisingly difficult.

7. Humming a familiar tune, hop to the left and right, mixing slow, large jumps with small faster ones.

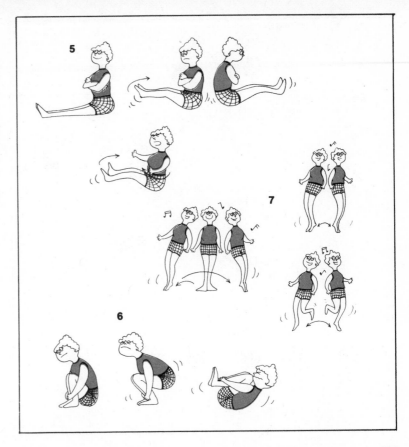

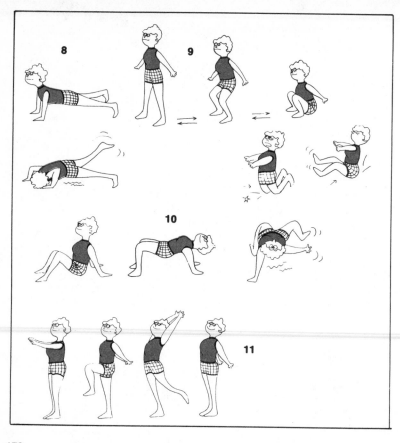

8. In a push-up position with legs spread, bend arms and touch forehead to right hand while lifting left leg high. Return to the original position. Then touch left hand while raising right leg. Touch both right and left hands 2 times if you are in your twenties, one time each if in your thirties, and either right or left just once if you are in your forties.

9. Stand with legs spread wide and lower yourself, keeping heels in place, until buttocks touch the floor, then rise again. There may be some women who at first find this difficult and fall onto their knees, but over time, this exercise will strengthen the legs and back. Do it 5 times.

10. Sit with hands on the floor behind, and arch back. Crab-walk, moving the arm and leg on the same side together. Be sure that you don't sag in the middle. It will take practice before you can move arms and legs together rhythmically. The exercise will strengthen the stomach muscles and give added endurance to the arms. Do 10 steps both right and left.

11. To cool down, do the following 8-count exercise: Lift arms in front; swing them down and back as you lift left knee; swing arms up high and left leg back, and arch your back; and return to the starting position. To the next 4 counts, repeat with the right leg. It may be difficult at first to coordinate arms and legs, but the emphasis should always be on the third and seventh counts. Do the exercise lightly, with a rhythmic bounce, 4 times.

12. Sitting on the floor with legs straight, rub, pound, and massage yourself all over—ankles, calves, thighs, stomach, neck, shoulders, and arms. Rub with palms until each spot is red and tingles.

Pointers for indoors

13. When cleaning house, use large strokes, whether with a dustrag, broom, or vacuum cleaner.

14. Do house chores briskly.

15. Keep good posture when cooking or doing dishes.

16. When picking something up off the floor, do not bend at the waist. Instead, keep back straight and bend at the knees.

17. After a bath or shower, dry yourself vigorously, using the towel as shown in Chapter 19.

Pointers for outdoors

18. Walk quickly, moving from the hips.

19. Walk at least 3 km (1.8 miles) every day.

20. Walk in 8 minutes what would ordinarily take 10.

21. When shopping, do not use elevators or escalators for up to four floors.

22. When waiting for a bus or subway, don't sit down.

23. Even if there is an empty seat on the bus or train, don't use it.

24. Don't wear high-heeled shoes.

25. When riding public-transportation vehicles, hold on to the strap or pole only lightly, if at all.

26. Play with your children outdoors as much as possible.

Chapter 35. Housework

The exercises in this chapter are good for any time of the day, but perhaps they are particularly applicable after supper.

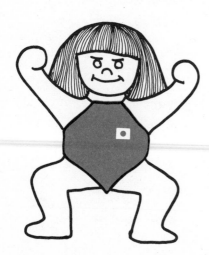

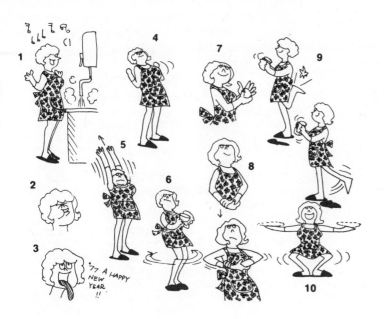

1. Whistle a melody.
2. Make funny faces.
3. Stick tongue out as far as possible.
4. Bend elbows, and arch back and chest.
5. Stretch arms over head as if to lift yourself off ground, neck scrunching up like a turtle's.
6. Swivel knees together without turning torso.
7. Massage palms and the bases of fingers.
8. Grasp right wrist firmly with left hand, and left wrist with right hand. Slowly slide hands all the way to shoulders; direction should be just wrist to shoulders.
9. Spread legs about 20 cm (8 inches) and swing legs straight back, one at a time. Also see if you can kick your behind with heel.
10. Spread legs slightly, with feet turned out and arms extended, imagining that you are balancing plates on hands. Bend at knees and breathe deeply.

Dishwashing exercises

These are exercises you can do while waiting for the dishpan to fill, or even while washing or drying dishes. They are recommended for straightening the spine, improving blood circulation, toning muscles, and increasing stamina.

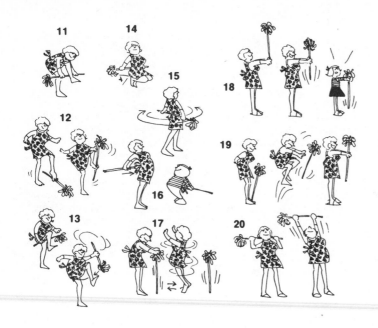

Using a duster

11. Hold duster horizontally in both hands and step over it and back, one leg at a time. Be as agile as possible.

12. Pick duster up with toes and pass it to hand. Repeat with other foot.

13. Standing erect, lift one knee and pass duster under thigh to other hand. As you are letting knee down, turn duster around. Lift other knee and pass duster back under. Learn to do this exercise rhythmically.

14. Hold duster in both hands behind back and do deep knee bends.

15. Hold duster in both hands behind back and twist torso to left and right. Do not allow feet to move.

16. Poke end of duster into small of back and arch backwards.

17. Stand duster on end and twirl yourself around before it falls over. Twirl to both left and right.

18. Hold duster vertically so that the end is at shoulder level. Drop and catch it before the duster part reaches shoulder level.

19. Stand with the end of duster between feet. Jump, tossing duster up, and catch it with one hand.

20. Hold duster in both hands behind neck across shoulders and lift it as if lifting a barbell. Let it down again as far below shoulders as you can.

These ten exercises are good also for children.

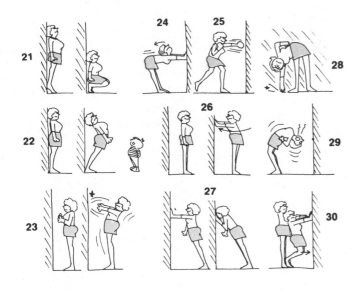

24. Face wall and bend forward with arms outstretched so that palms are flush against it. Lift head strongly up.

25. Shadowbox. Take care that you don't punch wall.

26. Stand with feet spread at shoulder width and with back to wall. Twist torso alternately to right and left, and place palms on wall.

27. Stand about 1 m (1 yard) from wall. Lean forward with one hand against wall. Bend elbow and touch head to hand. Straighten arm and repeat with other arm.

28. Stand with back against wall. Bend to left and touch left hand to floor. Repeat to right.

29. Stand with back to wall and hands at lower back. Bend over backward so that your head is at about waist level.

30. Stand with arms outstretched and palms against wall. Force knees forward.

Against a wall

21. Stand with back and heels flush against wall. Lift heels and then do deep knee bend.

22. Stand with back against wall. Push head against wall and arch body forward like a bow.

Chapter 36. Women's Sports Clinic

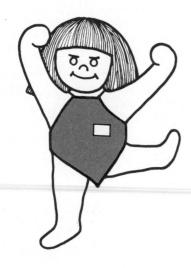

"Sports for anytime, anywhere, and anybody" is the motto of a broad movement to bring sports to the people. One part of that movement in a certain Japanese town was the women's sports clinic. This public service was not instituted as an end in itself, but rather with the hope that it would serve as a catalyst for the founding of various women's sports groups. The class would introduce a variety of activities and give basic instruction in them so that later the women could choose one to follow up.

The women's sports clinic is a ten-week course, meeting from 10:00 to 12:00 every Saturday morning. It has a capacity for fifty students. Each two-hour session covers a different sport or aspect of physical exercise, as follows:

Class 1: Traditional games and folk dances
Class 2: Physical fitness tests and beauty calisthenics
Class 3: Exercises with a volleyball
Class 4: Water games
Class 5: Badminton
Class 6: Tennis
Class 7: Ping-Pong
Class 8: Self-defense
Class 9: Western-style archery
Class 10: Physical fitness Olympics

In this chapter, I will focus on the activities of Class 7, which centers on Ping-Pong.

Running

Around the perimeter of the main floor of the local sports center, there is a 150-m (164-yard) track. For this class, the women run 30 seconds and walk 1 minute for about 15 minutes.

Physical fitness park

In front of the sports center, there is a physical fitness park that features a course along which there are various obstacles or tasks to be fulfilled. Some of these are shown in drawings 1-4. One of the advantages of such a course is that it can be used by both children and adults. Another attraction is its diversity of activities. The women spend 15 to 20 minutes on the course as part of their warm-ups.

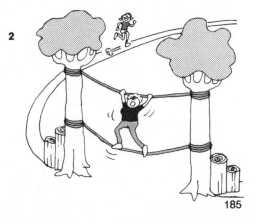

1

Fitness park

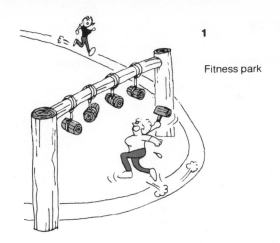

2

185

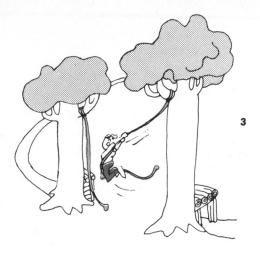

3

Ping-Pong

After exercising in the physical fitness park, the women came back inside. But before getting to the main order of the day, namely, Ping-Pong, they took a short break for refreshment and rest. Compared to their first class almost two months before, however, the women were less tired and out of breath. Clearly, their stamina level had risen.

Ping-Pong without tables

The women paired up and stood at the ends of courts measuring 1.5 m (5 feet) in width by 3 m (10 feet) in length, divided across the middle by a line. The first point to teach was the basic rules and how to hold the paddle in the handshake grip. Ten minutes were spent on this.

Each pair practiced batting a ball back and forth, always landing the ball in the opponent's court **(5).** They were instructed not to step inside the baseline, and were shown that accuracy was quite possible

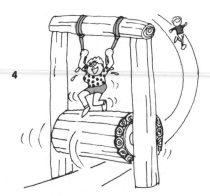

4

from a distance **(6).** They were also taught to swing with the elbow bent and relaxed, rather than tense and extended **(7).**

Setting up the tables

The women were taught how to set up a table and adjust the net properly. Four women were assigned to each table.

Basic strokes and volleying

The instructor then demonstrated the four basic strokes (drive and cut, forehand, and backhand), but explained that it would take time and practice before they could be mastered. First, he had the women stand close to the tables and volley with short shots. He told them to watch the ball carefully, no matter how fast it moved, and to notice the relationship between the feel of a shot and the action of the returned ball. Finally, he had the women back away from the edge of the table and practice longer shots, encouraging them to try for 10-stroke volleys.

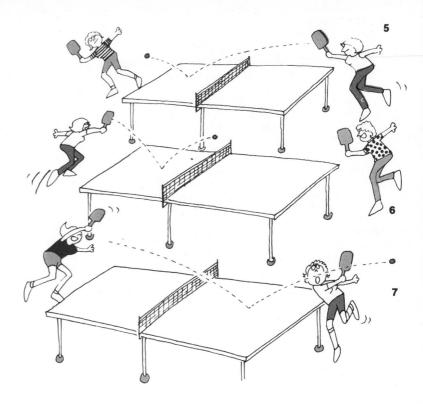

5

6

7

Cooling down

On the large mat in the training room, the women did the following cooling-down exercises:

8. Rolling: One partner lies on stomach with arms extended above head. The other bends over and slowly rolls her sideways to the other end of the mat. If she does this too fast, the first partner will become dizzy.

9. Rabbit hop: Crouching down, hop forward onto hands and push back to feet again.

10. Walking on knees: Move forward in a kneeling position with hands holding legs up by the ankles. It is surprisingly difficult to keep one's balance.

11. Seal crawl: Lie on stomach and pull yourself forward with arms.

12. Free-style beauty calisthenics: The class finished with a short period during which each participant did relaxing exercises of her own choice, such as sitting cross-legged and lying back, or doing bicycle pumping with legs in the air.

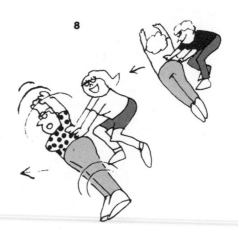

8

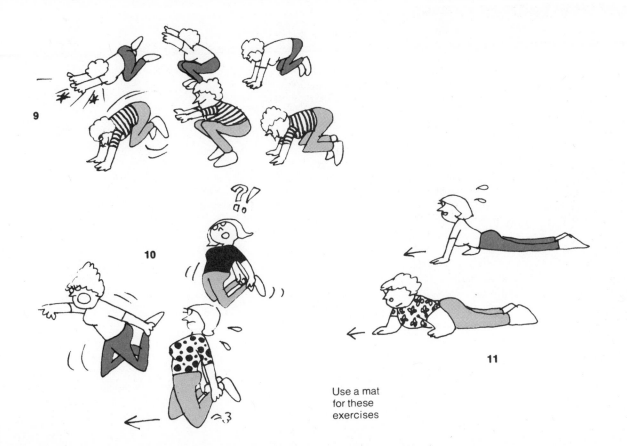

9

10

11

Use a mat
for these
exercises

189

Chapter 37. Jumping Rope

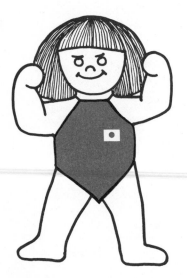

The last meeting of the ten-week women's physical fitness clinic focuses on exercises using a jump rope.

The instructor's plan for the class is as follows:

Warm-ups	(10 minutes)
Group exercises using one rope	(30 minutes)
Rope held taut (10 minutes)	
Rope twirled (20 minutes)	
Exercises in pairs using one rope	(5 minutes)
Relay races	(15 minutes)
Cooling down	(15 minutes)

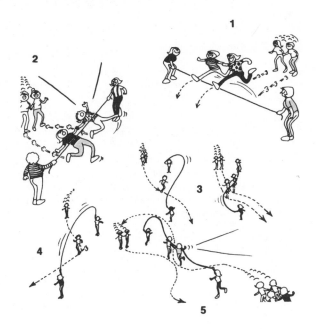

Warm-ups
Calisthenics

Group exercises using one rope
Rope held taut by two people

1. Begin with the rope held 30 cm (1 foot) off the floor. Each person jumps over twice. Then raise rope to 50 cm (20 inches). First, participants jump singly; then in pairs, holding hands; and the third time, in threes.

2. Next, with rope held 1 m (1 yard) high, each person bends backward and passes slowly underneath. The second time, rope is held at 80 cm (2 feet 7 inches) and participants pass under, holding hands in pairs. Finally, rope is held at 60 cm (2 feet).

Rope twirled by two people

3. Pass diagonally through swinging rope: This is the easiest approach, but it is important that the participants flow through quickly and without a break. Once they have gained the knack of going through one at a time, they may try it in pairs, holding hands, or with arms over each other's shoulders. One further variation is for the rope twirlers to change the pace of the rope on occasion.

4. Pass through rope in a hyperbola: Enter and exit on the same side of rope. This is not difficult to do singly, but when done in pairs, the inside person often gets caught in the rope. An interesting variation is to divide into two groups, one person from each group entering and exiting from opposite sides at the same time.

5. Pass through rope from head-on: Run through singly, in pairs and in fours, giving out healthy cheers on the way.

191

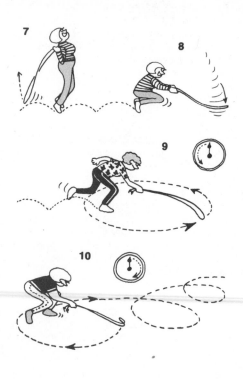

Exercises in pairs using one rope

6. One person swings the rope, the other enters, and the two jump together. Or the two jump side by side with arms over each other's shoulders, and twirl one end of the rope in their outer hands. Or, as a kind of rest, both face in the same direction, with one standing behind the other. The person in front walks with eyes closed, holding the rope as reins. The person in the rear tugs the rope on the right or the left to guide her. This is good training for the sense of balance and the sense of direction.

Jump-rope relay races

7. Hopping: Be sure that in the latter half of the run there are no unconscious in-between steps.

8. Hop and squat: Every third hop, land in squatting position. This is difficult for beginners because the speed of the rope must change.

9. Counterclockwise floor twirling: Hold both ends of rope in one hand and run, twirling it counterclockwise above floor. At first it is all right to insert extra steps, but toward the end each person should try to run smoothly, with one step for each twirl.

10. Clockwise floor twirling: Basically the same as above. To succeed, you must hold the rope in front of you, like a cotton-candy vendor.

Cooling down

For cooling down, the instructor passed out copies of the following "movement test," and had the participants take the test in pairs.

Ten-Part Movement Test

		1 Point	2 Points	3 Points
1. Back arching		Armpit height	Stomach height	Waist height
2. 360° body spin		Both right and left sloppy	Either right or left perfect	Both right and left perfect
3. Push-up position forward foot thrust		Can't do it at all	Can do it with a catch in the middle	Can do it perfectly
4. One-legged half knee bends		Can do one leg or other	Can do both 3 times	Can do both 5 times
5. Leg-spreading flexibility		Can touch head to floor	Can touch nose to floor	Can touch shoulder to floor
6. Standing from kneeling position		Can just barely stand	Can stand on one leg	Can jump to a stand
7. Leap and crawl (30 seconds)		8 times	14 times	Over 15 times
8. Backward broad jump		1/3 height	1/2 height	2/3 height
9. Hold ball between legs, toss in front, and catch		1 time	3 times in row	5 times in row
10. Hold ball behind back, toss over head, and catch		1 time	3 times in row	5 times in row

Total your points and find your grand total.

Chapter 38. Tennis Clinic

Although sports clinics and physical fitness classes have proliferated over recent years, there remains a strong misconception that sports clinics are fun, while physical fitness classes are tedious. In an attempt to correct this negative view, the physical fitness director in a certain Japanese city organized a three-month seminar for the city's sports instructors. After taking this seminar, a local tennis instructor decided to reshape the content of his classes. Let us look in this chapter at the program his women students now follow.

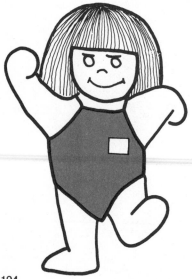

The class meets every Monday morning from 10:00 to 12:00, and lasts for ten weeks. There are forty in each class, applications having been accepted beginning one month in advance. There are also ten standby applicants in case one of the original forty drops out.

The following class plan is for the second meeting. Most of the students are beginners, but the basics had already been introduced in the first meeting. After the opening remarks by the instructor, participants do the following exercises.

Warm-ups
In pairs

1. Stand back to back with arms locked, walk sideways from one side of the court to the other, and then run back.

2. Play "scissors, paper, and stone." The loser carries the winner piggyback for 5 steps.

3. Stand 5 m (5 yards, 1 foot) apart, and bat the tennis ball back and forth on the bounce, using hands in place of rackets. At first, it is all right to stand directly facing each other, as in the illustration, so that the hand is almost pointing toward the partner when the ball is struck. Later, however, shift stance so that the body is at a right angle to partner and the hand meets the ball at a right angle.

Individual drills

4. Lay racket on ground and jump 3 times sideways back and forth across it. Then jump forward and backward 3 times across it.

5. Stand racket on head and try to twirl around once before it falls over. If you can do this twice in a row, you pass.

6. For footwork drills, practice a forehand swing with right foot extended, then left foot. Practice backhand swing with the same alternating footwork.

Main workout
Individual drills

7. Standing in place and holding racket in an Eastern grip **(8),** bounce ball on ground. Then bounce it while moving in a figure eight.

9. Practice bouncing ball on ground and then catching it with racket, alternating equally between backhand and forehand positions. Take care not to exert force when catching ball, or it will bounce away from you. Progress for beginners lies as much in learning the feel of receiving the ball as it does in actually hitting it. This exercise should help sensitize your touch.

In pairs

Stand facing each other in the same court, three steps inside the sidelines, and practice rallying on the bounce **(10).** As you return low balls, remember the feel of receiving. Return high balls with the sense of lightly stopping them. Make a 10-stroke rally your goal. Stay within the sidelines, and don't try to return poorly hit balls. The proper stance while waiting for a ball to be returned is with the free hand supporting the racket just below the frame **(11).** You should not let the racket hang loosely.

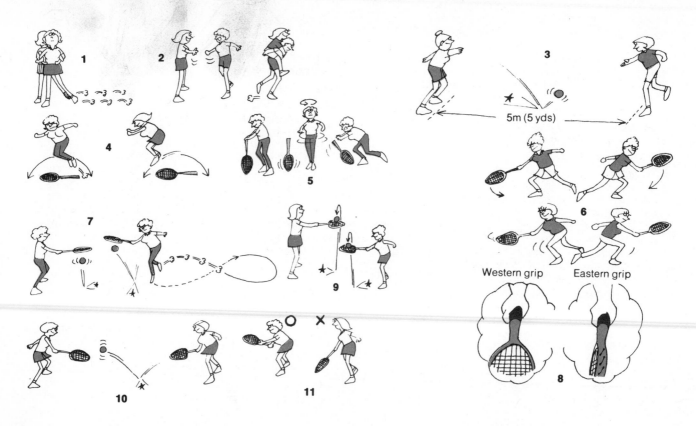

1

2

3

5m (5 yds)

4

5

6

7

8

Western grip   Eastern grip

9

10

11

Ground strokes

12. Two persons stand without rackets near the net. Behind them, near the baseline, two others stand with rackets. And in the opposite court two more stand, also with rackets. The two at the net throw balls one after another on one bounce to the pair in the opposite court, who then return the thrown balls to the far court, where they are retrieved. After the two have made 20 strokes, they rotate to the far court to chase balls, and the throwers take their places with rackets to hit them. While the women practice, the instructor moves from court to court, making suggestions and corrections.

Cooling down

13. Hold racket at both ends and jump over it as in jump rope.

14. Hold racket in right hand and swing it to the right. On return swing, pass it to the left hand and continue to the left. Pass it back to the right hand and repeat.

15. Lightly massage calves, buttocks, and the back of thighs with the frame of racket.

If one considers that basic physical fitness exercises can directly affect the sports reflexes and help speed the acquisition of athletic skills, one will have to agree that the above exercises, though not directly related to action on the court, are invaluable steps in the learning process.

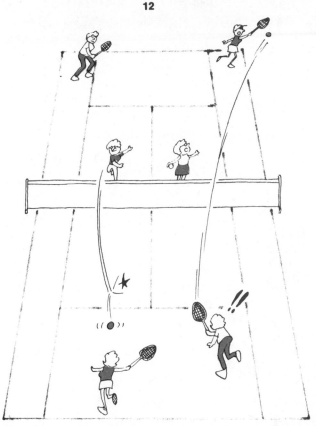

12

Chapter 39. Ping-Pong Clinic

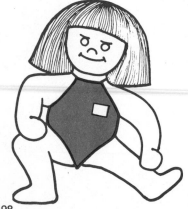

Each January, capitalizing on the buoyant spirits of the New Year and the communal sense of renewal which underpins that special season, the physical education council of a certain Japanese community sponsors a sports and physical fitness clinic for women.

This year the focus was on table tennis, or Ping-Pong. The popularity of the game, plus the feeling of many that they were overweight from all the holiday eating, brought an unusually large turnout. Capacity for the class was fifty, but because eighty people showed up for the first meeting, the event had to be moved from the table-tennis room to the main floor.

Outfitted in long-neglected training suits, the women began their individual warm-ups cheerfully and with friendly New Year's greetings (**1-4**). After the customary bending and stretching, the instructor started the women on a series of exercises using jump ropes.

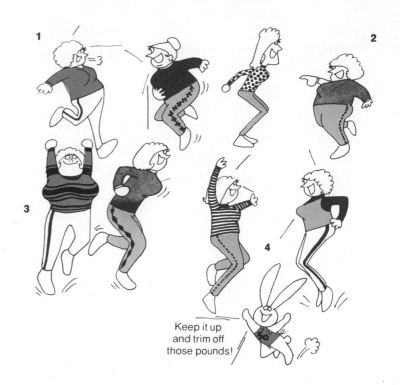

Keep it up
and trim off
those pounds!

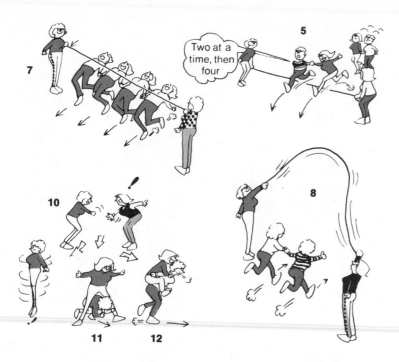

Two at a time, then four

Warm-ups

Group exercises using a long jump rope

5. Two people hold the rope taut at knee height. With a run of about 5 m (5 yards), the others jump over in pairs, holding hands.

6. Repeat in groups of four, again holding hands.

7. Rope is held at chest height, and participants pass under it in groups of four, bending backward.

8. Two swing the rope, while the others run straight through in pairs, holding hands.

9. Two swing rope, while the others run diagonally through in pairs, holding hands.

In pairs

10. Play "scissors, paper, and stone." Loser must jump and spin once around, sometimes to the right, sometimes to the left. This is done 10 times.

11. Play "scissors, paper, and stone." Loser must pass through winner's legs, without using hands for support. This is done 5 times.

12. Play "scissors, paper, and stone." Loser must carry winner piggyback for 7 paces. Continue until you have gone from one side of gym to the other and back. There is no regular alternation of carrier and carried. The loser always must carry.

Ping-Pong practice without tables

13. Each person bounces a ball on her paddle, aiming for a goal of 20 successive bounces. Use both forehand and backhand positions equally. Each is responsible only for her own ball, but must try to avoid the others. That's where much of the fun in this exercise lies.

14. Divide up into pairs, standing 5 to 7 m (5 to 8 yards) apart. Holding paddles in the handshake grip, volley on the bounce for 10 minutes, practicing the following combinations: forehand drives with backhand cuts; forehand drives with backhand drives; and forehand cuts with backhand cuts.

15. The instructor then had the women gather for a short and humorous demonstration of common mistakes and their correction. He discussed the serve, the correct body position for returns, and the mistake that many people make of extending the arm too far after making a return. During the instructor's presentation, some helpers set up a net-high veneer board across the length of the room. The women returned to their volleying, this time across the net, for 10 minutes. Although playing on the floor like this didn't change the need for correct style, it was easier to continue a long rally than when using a table. The women worked up a good sweat.

16. In pairs, at about 5 m (5 yards) apart, the women practiced volleying, without allowing the ball to touch the ground, for 5 minutes.

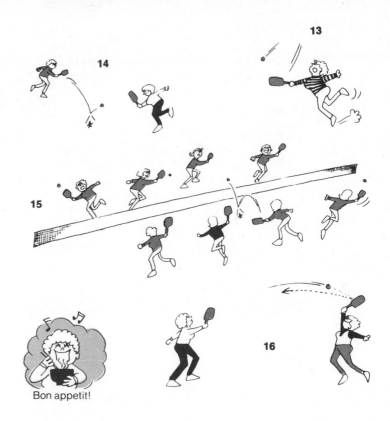

Bon appetit!

Using tables

17. The instructor showed the women how to set up the table and then had them volley with four at a table, using twenty tables in all, for 15 minutes.

18. Play doubles games of 11 points per game for 15 minutes.

Cooling down

19. Women massage each other in pairs.

20. Folk dancing.

21. In time to music, walk in a circle, balancing ball on paddle. Pass paddle to other hand, toss ball in air and catch it on paddle, and so on.

Since the day of this first class (January 11) coincided with a traditional observance called *o-shiruko* ("cutting of the rice cakes"), special refreshments were served after the women had changed. It had been prepared as a surprise for them by the physical education council in cooperation with a local women's group. This was a fitting and festive close to the gathering.

Chapter 40. Volleyball Clinic

Volleyball is the most popular sport among women in Japan and is always included in the programs set up by municipal physical education councils. The seven-week volleyball clinic is for beginners, who, it is hoped, will eventually serve as the nucleus for new neighborhood volleyball groups. Since the ultimate goal, of course, is physical fitness, the instructors hand out various pamphlets and leaflets about exercise and exercising techniques.

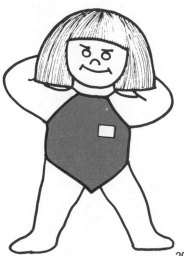

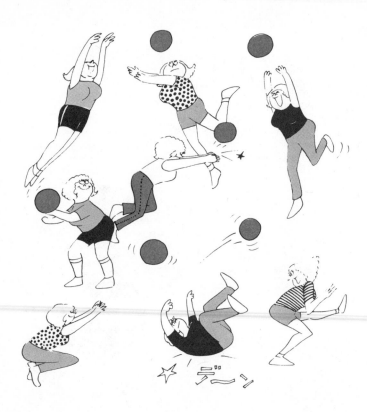

Today's class is being held on two courts at the municipal gymnasium. It is the third meeting of the clinic. Attendance has been very high, and today only two of the forty members are absent. Some mothers have left their young children in the nursery on the second floor. The fact that the city provides a full-time nursery service at the gymnasium is an indication of the importance with which physical fitness is regarded.

On the next pages are the instructor's class plan.

Warm-ups

Divide into groups of four, with pairs separated by the width of the court.

1. Volley, taking the ball on the bounce and returning it with underhand two-handed strokes. Start with small strokes, gradually using larger ones.

2. Volley, starting at 7 m (7 yards, 2 feet) apart. Partners must alternate in returning the ball. One bounce is allowed before returning, though it is not necessary. As players gain control, they may try to make it difficult for opponents.

3. Practice underhand serves between sidelines. The receiver should hold out hands as a mark for the server to hit. Receiver catches ball and returns it as a serve.

4. Volley, keeping the ball in the air as long as possible.

5. Volley at 5 m (5 yards, 1 foot) apart on the bounce. Try to make ball bounce at opponent's feet rather than in middle. One-handed overhand strokes are acceptable. It is also acceptable to use closed fists as well as open palms. The pace of such volleying will be faster, making for better exercise.

Individual drills

6. When reaching to return a ball which is falling short, it is natural to thrust one leg forward. For even greater reach, turn the rear foot over, as in the illustration. Practice walking about in this fashion.

7. Practice the tumbling return made famous by the Japanese women's volleyball team. Thrust right arm and leg diagonally forward as if to field a short-falling ball. Roll over on right shoulder and come to a standing position, ready to field another ball.

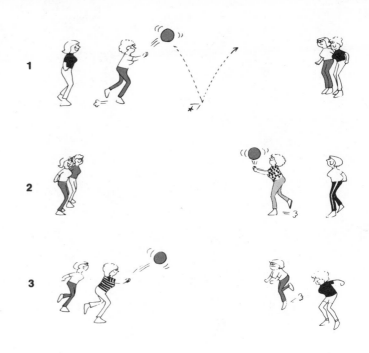

205

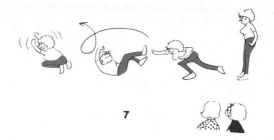

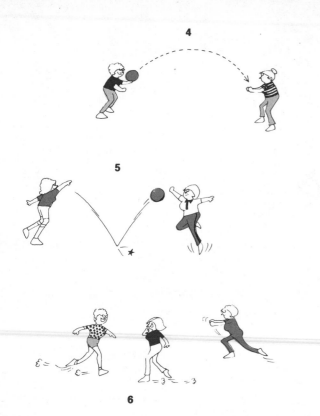

Game

Play 7-point games, six players on each side, using underhand serves. On each court, organize tournaments of five teams.

Cooling down

The instructor uses different cooling-down activities for each meeting.

Class 1: Exercises using the volleyball
Class 2: Two-handed passes
Class 3: Basics of passing and spiking; short games
Class 4: Serving practice; short games
Class 5: Spiking practice
Class 6: Game
Class 7: Game

Chapter 41. An Athletic Meet

In January, the graduates of a certain sports class for mothers held their fifth annual New Year's athletic meet. This event was so successful that it is worth a chapter.

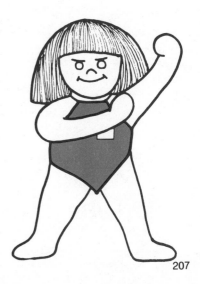

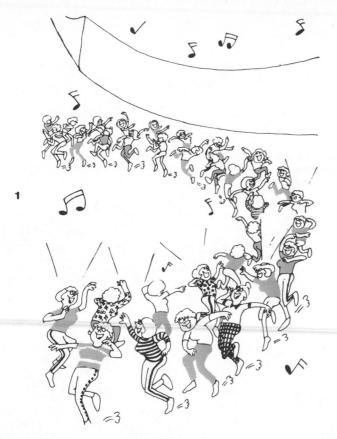

The graduates of this class now number about 250, and satellite classes have sprung up in surrounding areas, so the annual meet has become important. January was chosen because it is the time of year when people ordinarily are least inclined to be physically active. This is a way to renew old friendships and to encourage continued interest in physical exercise.

In late December, return postcards announcing the date, time, place, and registration fee (for refreshments) were sent out. About two hundred people, eighty-five percent of the total, responded with a desire to participate.

The program for the day was as follows:

1:00-1:30   Calisthenics
1:30-3:00   30-minute rotation periods between the "sweat shop," the "sports shop," and the pool
3:00-4:00   Socializing and refreshments

Calisthenics

1. The meet began with two large concentric circles of one hundred persons each. The circles moved in opposite directions, everyone exchanging New Year's greetings and dancing to the music of the *Awaodori*. As they say on the island of Shikoku, the home of the famous dance, "He who dances is a fool, but he who doesn't is even more a fool." After several minutes, the circles began to weave in and out of each other, gradually speeding up to a quick walk or a run near the end. This lasted 5 minutes.

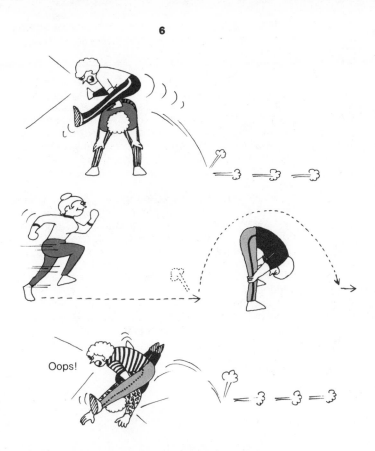

6

Oops!

2. Remaining in concentric circles, the participants held hands and danced to different music for 5 minutes.

3. The circles were then broken up, and each person did individual warm-up exercises of her own choosing—stretching, bending, and jumping—for 3 minutes.

4. Concentric circles were formed again. With legs spread at shoulder width, partners stood about 30 cm (1 foot) apart and tried to push each other off balance for 3 minutes.

5. The group divided into pairs. One partner of each pair sat with legs out on the floor while the other stood behind and massaged her neck, shoulders, and back for 3 minutes apiece.

6. Leapfrog: One partner bent down, hands on knees, and the other vaulted over from the side and then back again. Height was adjusted by spreading the legs wider or less wide. Positions were changed. The next time, the partner vaulted from the rear. The third time, one lay face down, with arms stretched above head. The other vaulted over by placing hands on partner's shoulders and lower back. This took 5 minutes.

7

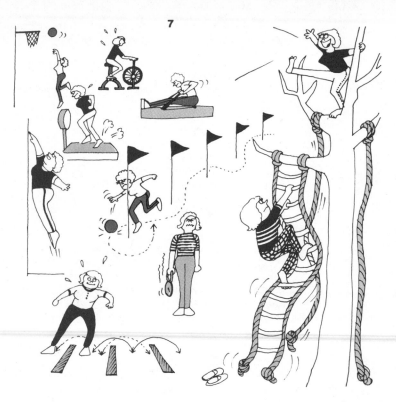

At this point, everyone divided into three groups, which rotated every 30 minutes between each of the following three areas.

Sweatshop

On the third floor of the building is a room equipped for various kinds of exercising **(7)**. At one end is a maple tree with ropes and a rope ladder hanging from its branches. There is a running meter, a rowing machine, a bicycle, and other exercising devices. There are places for the standing broad and high jumps. And there are instruments for measuring lung capacity, hand grip, and so on.

Sports floor

On the main floor there is ample space for two full basketball courts. For this meet, the space was used for one-bounce volleyball (without a net) and one-bounce Ping-Pong without tables **(8)**. The group was divided into pairs, which lined up 7 m (8 yards) apart. They began with volleyballs, hitting them back and forth on the bounce for 10 minutes. The women then continued in the same fashion, using Ping-Pong balls and paddles. Control is more difficult with a Ping-Pong ball than with a volleyball, so more footwork is necessary. This took 10 minutes.

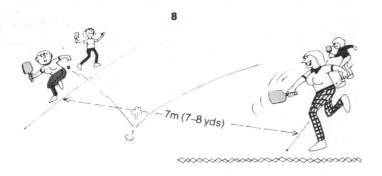

—— 7m (7–8 yds) ——

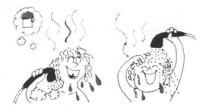

The pool

In the basement there is a 25- by 15-m (25- by 15-yard) pool and a smaller, shallow pool for children. Because bathing suits can be rented, those who did not bring their own could swim. For the first part of each swimming session the women swam about freely and enjoyed themselves. At the end, they divided into groups for a relay race, each person swimming 25 m (25 yards) holding a kickboard in front of her. This took 20 minutes.

After showering and drying their hair with the dryers provided, the women gathered in a meeting room to socialize.

Not only does this annual event renew old friendships and revitalize the spirit of physical fitness, it also provides an occasion for publicity. The local newspaper always covers the event and publishes at least one photo. This publicity draws new members into the continuing classes. In fact, some years, new classes had to be formed after the meet to accommodate new members.

One advantage in using the public facility is that a baby-care center is available, so that a mother can bring her child along with her.

PART V. FITNESS FOR THE FAMILY

Chapter 42. Fitness Begins at Home

There is a Japanese proverb which says: "The spirit of the child of three will live to be a hundred." Whether or not this is a version of the saying, "The child is father of the man," it is certainly as valid in the East as its Western counterpart is in the West. If a child is brought up in a home which is racked with tension, its personality will be adversely affected. And if its parents are uninterested in sports or exercise, very likely the child will be adversely influenced for life. It is therefore the duty of the parent to provide a health-giving atmosphere in which the child may grow up.

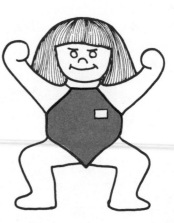

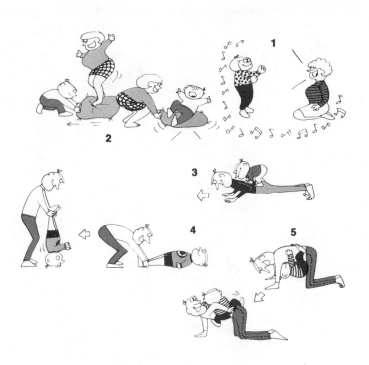

Play with your child at least 10 minutes each day

1. Sing songs. Play song games. If you can, provide instrumental accompaniment. Add movement to songs.

Once each day, satisfy your child's spirit of adventure

2. Have him stand on a cushion and see if he can keep his balance as you pull it gently this way and that. Then, after you've made sure the area is safe, have him try to upset you as you stand on the cushion.

3. Turtle push-ups: Slowly do push-ups with child kneeling on your back.

4. Foot-hanging: Have child lie on his back. Pick him up by the ankles and gently swing him back and forth once or twice.

5. Monkey: The parent kneels on all fours and the child hangs around the parent's belly. From that position, the child then clambers up onto parent's back. The first few times, the parent may have to help him.

6. Mighty Mouse: a) The parent stands behind the child, picks him up by the waist, lifts him feetfirst overhead, and gently lets him down behind. *b.)* Then the parent sits on the floor and has the child hold onto the parent's legs. With hands at the child's waist, the parent slowly rolls backward, lifting the child up with the legs and flipping him over onto feet just above parent's head.

Sports inside the house

7. Batting practice with a rolled newspaper and a Japanese paper balloon (or a regular balloon).

8. Swordplay: Have a fencing match with rolled newspapers or with rug beaters. Tie pillows to head and stomach for protection.

9. Sumo (Japanese wrestling): Child stands, parent squats. Or parent wrestles on one leg.

10. Upside-down bowling: Stand back to back some distance from each other and bend over. Roll a ball back and forth between legs.

For your information

• A three-year-old child needs twelve hours of sleep each day.

• A two- or three-year-old child normally takes 25 to 30 breaths per minute.

• Normal handgrip for a six-year-old is 14 kg (31 pounds) for a boy, 12 kg (26 pounds) for a girl.

• A four-year-old's pulse should be about 100 per minute, a ten-year-old's should be 90.

• A six-year-old's lung capacity is 1,000 ml (60 cubic inches).

• The normal blood pressure of a three-year-old is 80/65. A ten-year-old's is 95/70.

214

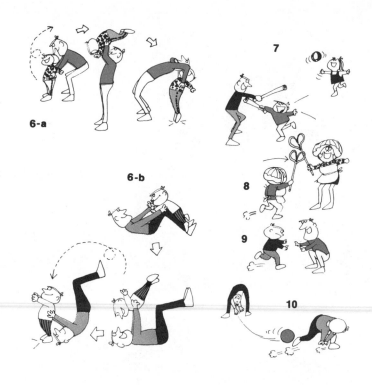

6-a

6-b

7

8

9

10

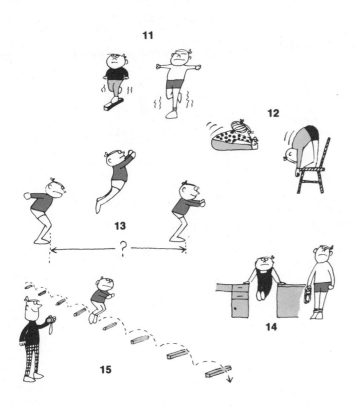

A physical fitness test for children

11. Balance: How long can the child stand one-footed on a narrow block 3 by 3 by 30 cm (1 1/2 by 1 1/2 by 12 inches)? A child six or over should do the same test on the floor but with eyes closed.

12. Flexibility: Have the child sit on floor with legs stretched out and bend forward. Measure how far fingers extend beyond heel. A six-year-old should stand on a chair and bend down. Measure how far his fingers reach below the seat of the chair.

13. Leg power: Measure length of child's standing broad jump.

14. Strength: How long can the child support himself between two desks? If he is six or older, test him with a hand dynamometer.

15. Agility: Lay ten toy blocks 50 cm (20 inches) apart, and time how long the child takes to hop between them.

The following charts give the average results of boys and girls of different ages in the above five-part test. How well did your child do? A simpler, more basic physical fitness test for children is given in the next chapter to help guide you in planning your children's activities.

Standard Physical Fitness Test Results—Boys

Age	Balance (seconds)	Flexibility (inches)	Leg Power (inches)	Strength	Agility (seconds)
4-4¹/₂	3	1¹/₂-2¹/₃	36	21-41 seconds	13-10
4¹/₂-5	4	2-2³/₄	36	32-63	12-9
5-5¹/₂	5	1¹/₂-2³/₄	41	43-88	11-9
5¹/₂-6	6	1¹/₂-3¹/₈	41	49-130	9-7
6	15	2-3¹/₈	47	22-24 lbs	8-6
7	20	2¹/₃-3¹/₂	52	26-29	—
8	26	2¹/₂-4	56	29-33	—
9	32	2³/₄-4¹/₃	60	33-37	—
10	39	3¹/₈-4³/₄	64	37-42	—

Standard Physical Fitness Test Results—Girls

Age	Balance (seconds)	Flexibility (inches)	Leg Power (inches)	Strength	Agility (seconds)
4-4¹/₂	3	3¹/₂-4¹/₃	34	30-63 seconds	14-9
4¹/₂-5	4	3¹/₈-4³/₄	34	32-73	13-9
5-5¹/₂	5	2³/₄-4¹/₃	40	42-100	11-8
5¹/₂-6	6	2³/₄-4¹/₃	40	55-105	9-7
6	18	2³/₄-4	44	20 lbs	8-6
7	20	2³/₄-4	50	22-24	—
8	22	3¹/₈-4¹/₃	53	26-29	—
9	25	3¹/₂-4³/₄	56	29-33	—
10	29	4-5¹/₂	59	33-37	—

Average Physical Development Statistics

Age	MALE			FEMALE		
	Height (inches)	Weight (pounds)	Chest (inches)	Height (inches)	Weight (pounds)	Chest (inches)
3-3$\frac{1}{2}$	37	31	20$\frac{1}{3}$	36$\frac{2}{3}$	29	19$\frac{7}{8}$
3$\frac{1}{2}$-4	38$\frac{1}{2}$	33	20$\frac{2}{3}$	38	31	20$\frac{1}{8}$
4-4$\frac{1}{2}$	40	35	21	39$\frac{1}{4}$	33	20$\frac{3}{8}$
4$\frac{1}{2}$-5	41	37	21$\frac{1}{3}$	40$\frac{1}{2}$	35	20$\frac{3}{4}$
5	43$\frac{1}{3}$	41	22	42$\frac{7}{8}$	40	21$\frac{1}{2}$
6	45$\frac{1}{5}$	44	22$\frac{1}{2}$	44$\frac{3}{4}$	43	21$\frac{7}{8}$
7	47$\frac{1}{4}$	49	23$\frac{1}{4}$	47	48	22$\frac{2}{3}$
8	49$\frac{1}{3}$	55	24$\frac{1}{5}$	49$\frac{1}{8}$	54	23$\frac{2}{3}$
9	51$\frac{1}{3}$	61	25$\frac{1}{8}$	51$\frac{1}{3}$	61	24$\frac{1}{2}$
10	53$\frac{1}{3}$	68	26	53$\frac{3}{4}$	68$\frac{1}{2}$	25$\frac{2}{3}$

Chapter 43. For Your Children

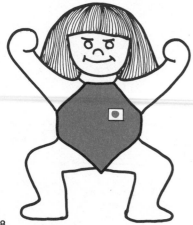

Children have a voracious appetite for both knowledge and physical activity. But while the appetite for knowledge is glutted in an information overload, the need for physical exercise is frustrated by cramped living quarters, congested traffic conditions, and the intense academic pressure which begins in elementary school. This is unhealthy both spiritually and physically. It is true that there has been a renewed awareness of the importance of preschool education, but within that context, it is crucial that we reexamine our attitude toward the early physical development of our children.

Unfortunately, parents too often indulge their own competitive spirit when watching their child's development. As soon as the infant starts to crawl, they urge him or her to stand. No sooner can the child stand than they want him or her to walk. And later, in sports, they want only that their child be better than the others.

To sow the seeds of true delight in physical exercise, it is necessary first to ensure that the environment permits fulfillment of the child's natural need for exercise.

Test your very young child's fitness

The Kraus-Weber basic physical fitness test will help you to know your very young child's strength. Most children will be able to do all of the six tasks. If your child is unable to do two or more, however, he will need your help to keep up with the other children. You can help him overcome this deficiency by carefully leading him through a program of home exercises. Take notice of the movements and facial expressions of the child as he or she does the following tasks.

Kraus-Weber Test

1. Can the child do a sit-up with hands clasped behind head and knees flexed?

2. Can the child do a sit-up with knees straight?

3. Can the child lift one leg at a time so that toes are one foot from the floor, holding it to the count of 10?

4. Can the child lie face down, while you hold his ankles, and lift chest, shoulders, and head to the count of 10?

5. Can the child lie face down and lift one leg at a time to the count of 10 without bending the knee?

6. Can the child stand and touch the floor with hands without bending knees?

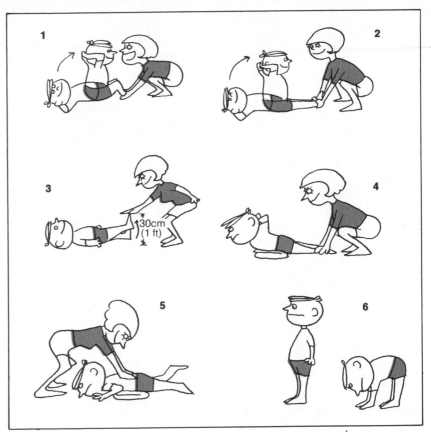

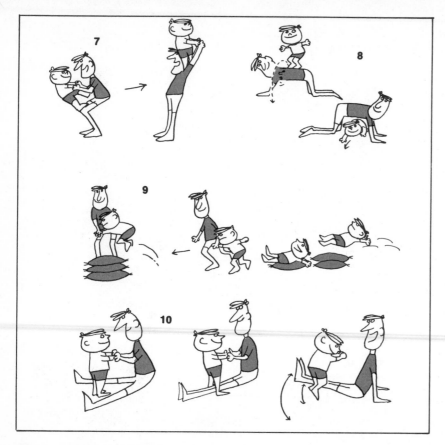

Play with your child

Ten minutes of physical play with your child each day will bring many benefits. It will enhance the parent-child relationship; it will enhance home life; and it will give you yourself exercise. Nine exercises are illustrated here (**7–15**), but it is easy to think up many others.

Consider also the objects which our children use in play. Playground equipment is the same everywhere—solid and permanently in place. But there is no reason why children today can't be happy with traditional games and playthings such as hopscotch, jump rope, and stilts.

Help your child learn to love nature. Running on an open beach, walking in the countryside, and sled riding in the snow are activities which will contribute significantly to a child's growth and will leave him with happy memories. And if you take walks regularly as a family, have a footrace along the way; if you play kickball or other outdoor games near your home, think how much greater the pleasure will be when you are able to get away for an outing in the country.

If you as a parent are aware of the importance of physical fitness and take active steps to promote it for both you and your child, that child will follow your example and will naturally grow strong and healthy.

As I have said, the child's fitness depends on the environment in which he grows. But by environment, I mean not only material surroundings or playthings. More important is the spiritual and physical guidance of the parent. Raising a child without such proper guidance is like plowing the field but forgetting to sow the seed. Leisure time directed toward physical and spiritual fitness should be one of the most important pillars in the home education of your child.

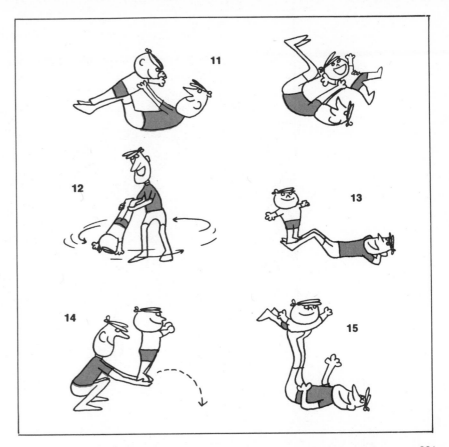

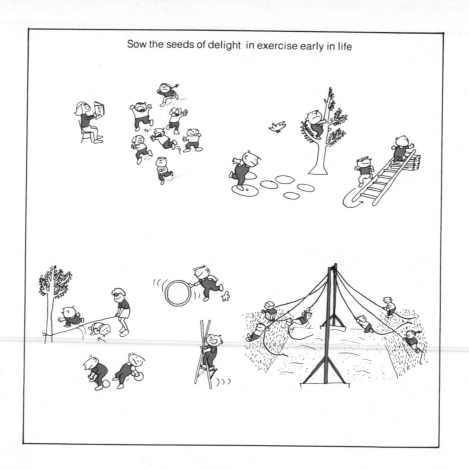

Sow the seeds of delight in exercise early in life

Chapter 44. In the Nursery School

Miss Ashizawa taught in an urban nursery school. During the day she was totally responsible for the care of twenty children. She was good at her job, working selflessly and caught up wholeheartedly in the work. One day, however, she began to notice that her children were not as spirited and energetic as before. She thought that probably this was a result of outside pressures, such as private lessons of various sorts after school.

Of course, every day in the nursery school the children participated in different physical activities, such as rhythm exercises with tambourine and castanets, and playing outdoors on the jungle gym and slide. But Miss Ashizawa realized that a better-organized program was needed to support the strains under which the children lived.

She tried a variety of approaches over the course of half a year, receiving not a little criticism from overprotective mothers who worried that the children would be too tired for other things, or that they might injure themselves. Contrary to this concern, however, the children flourished. Their faces seemed brighter than ever, and eventually the parents became convinced of the value of the new approach.

Miss Ashizawa's greatest success was a parent-child winter sports outing which she arranged. For three days and two nights, the group stayed at a northern ski resort. The experience of sliding down the slopes on squares of vinyl, parents and children together, was exhilarating. (See also Chapter 56.)

From then on, Miss Ashizawa's physical fitness program was given the full support of all. Clearly, it was helping the children develop not only in body, but in mind and spirit as well.

Let us look at the exercise program for a typical day at Miss Ashizawa's nursery school.

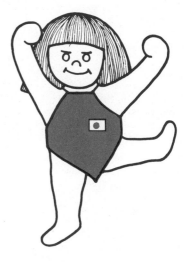

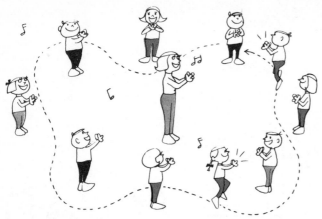

2. Ball bouncing: Still in two circles, the children are each given a ball and instructed to perform certain tasks with it in time to a song which everyone sings. The tasks include throwing and catching the ball, catching it on one bounce, bouncing it under a lifted leg, bouncing it with one hand, and bouncing it with both hands.

1. Clapping and skipping: Make two large circles of ten children each. While everyone sings and claps in time, two children in each group skip around the circle, weaving in and out of the others.

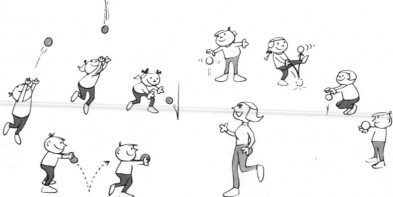

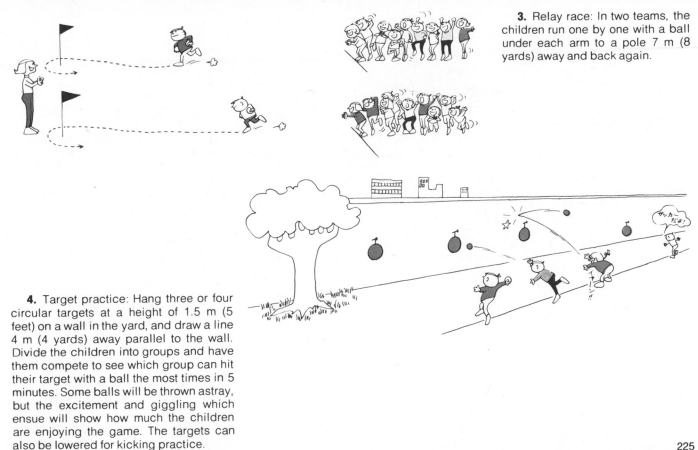

3. Relay race: In two teams, the children run one by one with a ball under each arm to a pole 7 m (8 yards) away and back again.

4. Target practice: Hang three or four circular targets at a height of 1.5 m (5 feet) on a wall in the yard, and draw a line 4 m (4 yards) away parallel to the wall. Divide the children into groups and have them compete to see which group can hit their target with a ball the most times in 5 minutes. Some balls will be thrown astray, but the excitement and giggling which ensue will show how much the children are enjoying the game. The targets can also be lowered for kicking practice.

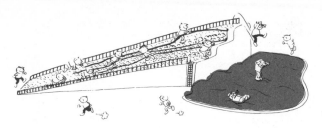

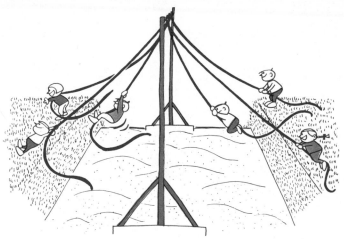

5. Rock climbing: There is a concrete ramp at a grade of about 20 with rocks of various sizes fixed into it. The end of the ramp is divided into three levels, ranging from 1.5 m (5 feet) at the highest to 80 cm (2 feet, 8 inches), from which the children can jump into a sand area at the base. There are ropes attached at the top with which the children can pull themselves up the ramp. The teacher must tell each child from which height he or she can safely jump. Once that is decided, the children will watch out for themselves. This is an activity which they especially love. And with the proper guidance, it is perfectly safe.

6. Tarzan: This particular nursery school has no swing. In its place, there is a crossbar from which ropes are suspended. Below, there is a sandpit, banked by turf. The children swing from one bank to the other, pretending they are Tarzan swinging from tree to tree. As they play, of course, they increase the strength in their arms.

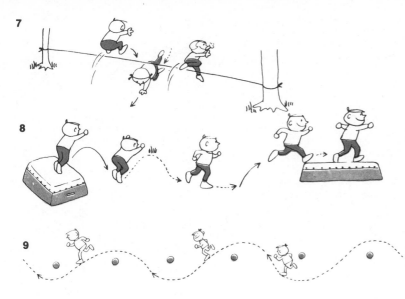

Miss Ashizawa has devised many other exercise activities (**8** and **9,** for example), but this was enough for one day, so she had the children return to the classroom, holding balls high over their heads and twisting their bodies to the right and left as they marched in.

Miss Ashizawa's ingenuity was praised by the parents, and many of her ideas were adopted for play at home. Particularly impressive, however, was her wisdom in having showers installed so that the children could wash and change clothes before continuing the rest of the school day. One smiles just to think of the happy children standing under the shower after their invigorating exercise.

One might think at first that such aftercare is an unnecessary luxury, but without it the value of the exercise period is greatly reduced. It is to Miss Ashizawa's credit that she recognized this and took the initiative in requesting the shower facilities.

The parents were all extremely happy with the results of Miss Ashizawa's physical fitness campaign. The children were healthier, and more alert and responsive at home. They were clearly on the road to developing into well-rounded individuals.

7. Rubber band jumping: Attach a long rubber string between two trees or poles at a height of 20 cm (8 inches) which the children can jump over and crawl under.

Chapter 45. A Nursery School Teacher's Guide

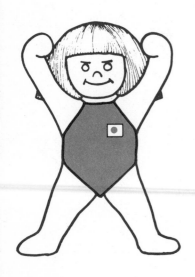

It is not only adults in our modern age who have increasingly fewer opportunities to use their bodies. Children also have lost touch over time with the wealth of games and activities which children of the past once enjoyed. The traditions, the customs, and the creativity of a day gone by have been caught up and crushed in the great cogwheel of our materialistic civilization. In this closed-room society, children for whom physical play was at one time a way of life now sit glued to the television set, or fiddle with "educational" toys. Like a dog tied to his doghouse, they have had the natural desire for physical activity domesticated out of them.

With the increasing emphasis on the importance of early education, more and more children are being sent to nursery schools and other educational facilities. One could take a superficial view of this and criticize the parents for shirking a personal responsibility in their child's development. More realistically, however, our concern should be directed at the schools, and at whether they are providing a structure within which the child's need for physical activity can be satisfied. All too often, these schools have only limited space. The challenge presented to the teacher is a great and important one indeed.

Let us consider in this chapter some ideas with which this challenge can be met.

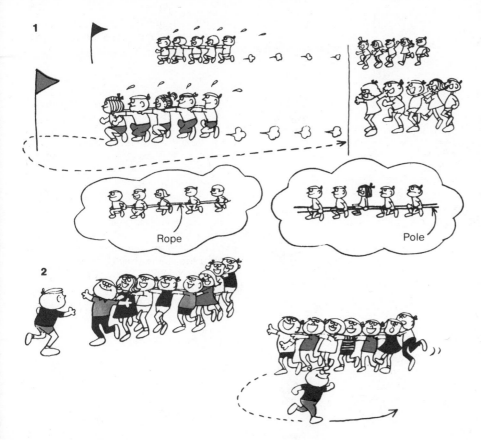

Rope

Pole

Reintroduction of traditional play activities

1. Caterpillar race: The children are divided into teams of five. Each child crouches down with his hands on the shoulders of the child in front. The teams race like caterpillars over a fixed course. The course may be any length or shape. If it is too difficult for the children to maneuver with hands on shoulders, they may hold on to ropes or bamboo poles.

2. Child-catching: One child in a group of from five to ten is designated a goblin; another, the protecting parent; and the rest, children. The children line up with each child's hands on the shoulders of the one in front, the child at the head of the line being the protecting parent. He waves his hands to scare off the goblin when the goblin attacks. The children should be instructed to hold on tightly to the one in front so that the line does not break. In a variation on this game, the line itself is a dragon. The child at the head of the line cries, "I'm going to eat you up," breaks away, and runs around to catch the end of the line, which of course tries to escape.

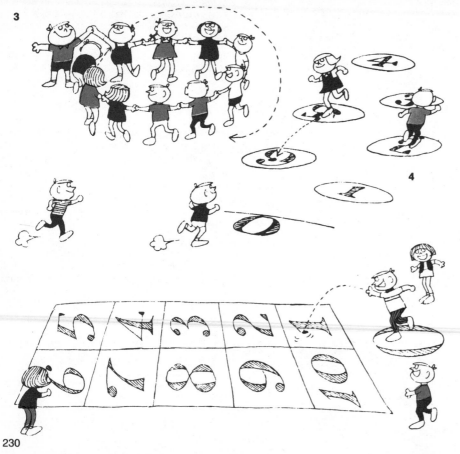

3. Snake in the hole: The children hold hands in a single line. The first two in the line raise their hands, and the rest of the line, starting at the other end, goes underneath.

4. Japanese hopscotch: The game is started, as shown in the drawing, by throwing a stone from the starting circle into the first division. Hopping on one foot, the player follows the stone, kicks it into the next division, hops after it, and so on. When he reaches the last division, he kicks the stone out, hops to the starting circle, and begins again, this time throwing the stone into the second division and following it around. If he can do this all the way to the tenth division, he is the winner.

The game may be made easier by decreasing the number of divisions; it may be made more difficult by separating the divisions and making them circular. For older children, a rule can be made that only one kick is allowed for each division. There are numerous other variations which can be invented.

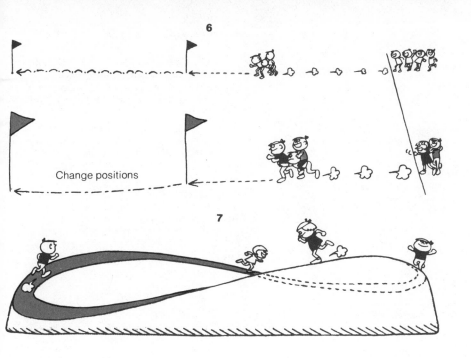

6

Change positions

7

5. Goblin: In the simplest form of this game, one child is the goblin until he catches another, who in turn becomes the goblin. In a variation, the caught child becomes a goblin and joins forces with the first, until all have become goblins. In yet another variation, certain spots may be designated as "safe" for children, where they cannot be caught.

6. Horse racing: A relay race in groups of three.

7. Playing and running liberate the rhythm and excitement which is natural in children, but which today is so often pent up and frustrated. Such activities are effective not only during school hours, but also will carry over into the child's free time, making physical exercise an integral part of his or her life.

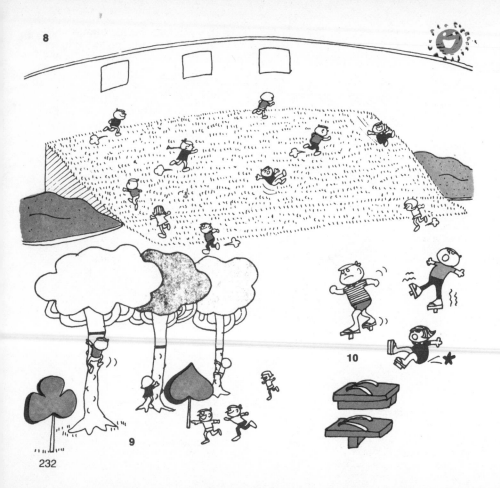

Improvement of playground facilities

In the small yards which nursery schools have for outdoor play areas, ordinary playground equipment such as swings and slides is all too common. These areas could be more effectively utilized by thinking in three-dimensional, rather than just two-dimensional terms. For example, a small but hilly running course or a play slope could be constructed, as shown in illustrations **8** and **9**. Another idea is to have the children walk around wearing one-toothed *geta* (Japanese wooden clogs which usually have two teeth) to help improve their sense of balance (**10**). An American nursery-school director suggests substituting stilts, or even empty coffee cans for this balancing exercise.

There is a Japanese proverb which says that new ideas can be found by examining the old. This is certainly true with ideas about physical fitness. Our children would benefit greatly by the restoration of the games of the past.

9

10

Chapter 46. Mother and Young Child Fitness Clinic

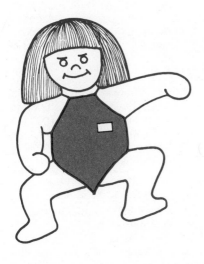

Mr. Motoyoshi, an experienced physical fitness instructor, was requested to lead a clinic for mothers and children in the exercise room of a certain young men's association building. The class was to consist of thirty mothers and their three-year-old children. The meeting time was from 11:00 to 12:00 every Tuesday morning.

All too often such classes tend to use the child as an object of exercise for the mother, but Mr. Motoyoshi was well known for giving equal emphasis to both parent and child. His first class is described below.

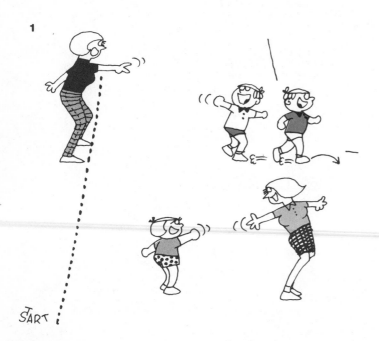

1

START

Warm-ups

The class began with each parent-child couple holding hands and greeting nearby couples with a hearty "Good morning."

1. Scissors, paper, and stone race: Parent and child play "scissors, paper, and stone" to determine who moves and how far along a 30-m (33-yard) course. If the winner wins with scissors, he moves 3 paces, and if he wins with paper or stone, he moves 6 paces.

2. Piggyback or pushing: If the child crosses the finish line first, the parent must carry him piggyback for 10 paces, with a spin after 5 paces. If the parent crosses first, the child must push the parent back for 10 paces, the parent providing a suitable amount of resistance.

Playing with Mother

3. Let's become a bird or animal: Parent and child face and say, "Here comes a butterfly," and the child circles the mother while imitating a butterfly. Then the child says, "It's your turn," and the mother circles the child, imitating a butterfly in a different way. Continue with other imitations. The child should always be first, so that his imagination is not constricted by seeing what his mother does.

4. Swordplay: Mother sits on floor and child stands, each holding in right hand a rolled newspaper as substitute for a bamboo kendo fencing stick. They play "scissors, paper, and stone" with their left hands. The winner of each throw gets to strike the other once with the newspaper sword. The loser holds up sword in defense.

2

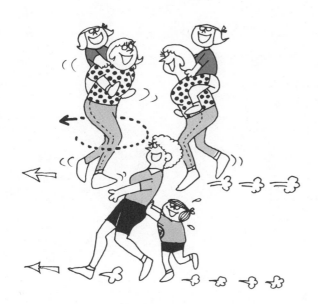

3

4

5

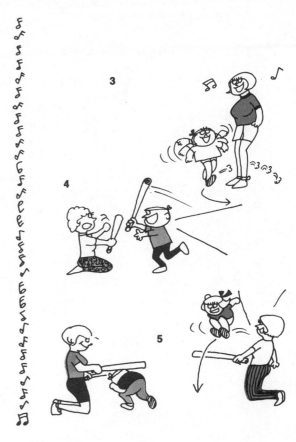

235

5. Jumping and ducking: The mother kneels with one rolled sheet of newspaper in each hand. These are held at different levels, so that the child can jump over one and duck under the other. The heights may be changed, sometimes the right higher, sometimes the left. Finally, both are held low at the same height and the child does a standing broad jump over both.

Playing with a ball

6. Through the hoop: Two parent-child couples work together, one holding a Hula-Hoop, the other throwing a ball through it. Change positions after 1 minute.

7. Ball kicking: Ten parent-child couples hold hands in a circle and kick a ball about. If the ball stops short of the other side, the circle must sag to kick it back.

8. Ball relay: The thirty couples are divided into three teams—red, white, and blue. The ten couples on each team divide into two groups and line up facing one another 20 m (22 yards) apart. Parent and child in each couple run together with a ball. The child throws it in the air, catches it, and then passes it to his mother. She throws it in the air from behind her back so that it goes over her head and catches it in front. She then passes it back to her child, and so on.

9. The wait-wait ball relay: With the same team arrangement as above, the ball this time is rolled from parent through legs of the child waiting in front. The child catches it and waits until his mother runs in front and opens her legs wide so that he can roll the ball between them.

Cooling down

10. Don't fall off: The mother lies face down, with legs slightly apart. The child walks on top of her, beginning with her legs, trying not to fall off.

11. Let's dance: Everyone dances to whatever music is popular.

The sight of all these sweating mothers and children was the picture of health itself, and also of happiness, for the experience opened doors to valuable new friendships. After everyone had rested awhile, a light lunch was served. Then those who wished went together to the nearby gymnasium so that the children could play in the children's swimming pool.

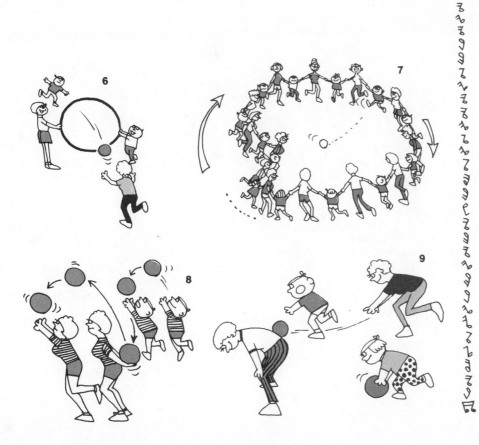

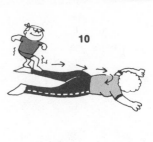

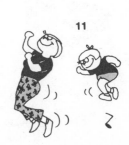

Chapter 47. Child Safety

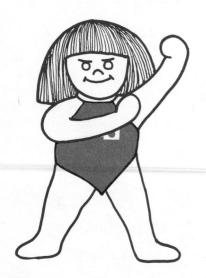

The beginning of the Japanese school year is a time of pride and excitement for those youngsters who are entering the first grade. For their parents, however, it is an anxious time, especially in the big cities, with the high incidence of accidents and injuries.

A certain district in Tokyo sponsored a physical fitness for safety clinic for parents with children who were about to begin school. Of course, all schools give instruction in traffic safety, but these programs make no sense unless the child's body can adapt. The idea of the clinic was to start the parent and child on a home program to improve the child's agility, coordination, and strength, and at the same time, to impress on the parent the importance of physical fitness to the child's safety and well-being. There is a tendency for parents to blame school authorities for an accident to their child, and sometimes the parent's claim may be justified. But the parents must realize that they too have an important responsibility in ensuring the child's safety, part of which lies in providing for his physical fitness.

The clinics were held in conjunction with physical checkups at the various elementary schools on the day before school began. At each elementary school, four fifty-minute clinics were given, with fifty parent-child couples participating in each. Physical checkups were given immediately afterwards. After brief introductory remarks by the school principal, two veteran physical education instructors began the class on the wall-to-wall gymnastic mats.

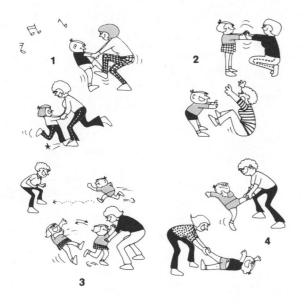

Mother-child competition

1. Foot stomping (1 minute): Mother and child face and hold hands. When music begins, they try to step lightly on each other's toes.

2. Pushing (3 minutes): Mother crouches in front of child. They put palms together and try to upset each other's balance.

3. Collision (5 minutes): Mother braces herself, and child runs into her. She gently pushes the child away.

4. Hop-hop (5 minutes): Mother lifts one of child's legs to his waist level and moves it gently about while child hops to keep balance. Pushing backward is the most difficult maneuver for the child to cope with.

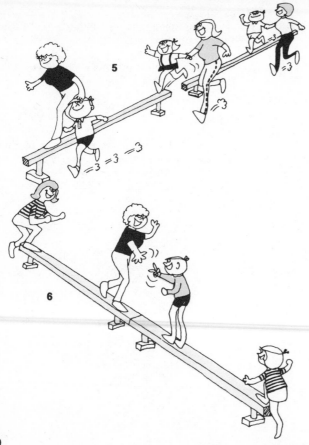

Playing with Mother

5. Horizontal-bar walking (5 minutes): Children walk along two horizontal bars which are 2 m (2 yards) long and 40 cm (16 inches) high. The two bars are set end to end, separated by 40 cm (16 inches), so that the child must jump to cross from one to the other. Mother walks along holding child's hand. When the mother walks on bar, she should place hand on head of child walking beside her. The third time around, the children may run lightly.

6. Horizontal-bar race (5 minutes): Two horizontal bars are joined. Parents line up at one end, children at the other. At a signal ("ready, go"), parent and child mount the bars at opposite ends and move toward center. At the spot where they meet, they play "scissors, paper, and stone." The loser dismounts from the bar, and the two race to see which can reach the other's starting point first. If parent or child falls from the bar either before or after playing "scissors, paper, and stone," it automatically becomes the next couple's turn.

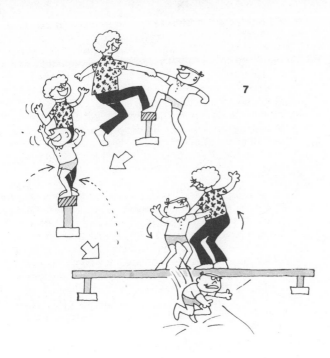

7. King of the horizontal bar (5 minutes): Mother and child face, with the horizontal bar between them. They hold right hands and place their right feet (outside of foot to outside of foot) on the bar. At the count of three they stand on the bar, let go their hands, and try to force the other off by pushing at the back. Out of 10 tries, whoever is successful most often is the winner.

7

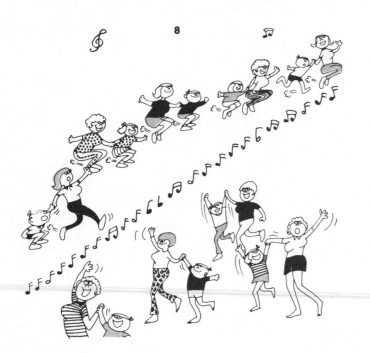

Onward with Mother (3 minutes for each exercise)

8. Mother-and-child pairs hold hands and parade around room to march music. When the instructor calls out "Red light!" everyone immediately stops, and when he calls "Green light!" everyone keeps marching. Next, they practice doing the opposite of what the instructor calls. When he calls "Right," everyone holds up his left hand, and when he calls "Left," everyone holds up his right hand. This is complicated by the fact that parents and children are holding hands, so only outer right or left hand is held up.

To conclude the class, one of the instructors gave a short summary of the lesson he hoped the children, and especially the parents, would take home with them. Cautioning the child to observe safety rules is important, he said, but unless such cautions also guide his physical responses, they can have the negative effect of making the child passive and overprotected. The instructor urged the mothers to encourage their children's physical development so that they could get by in life with only shin bruises and avoid the major bone-breaking calamities.

Chapter 48. Teaching Children to Swim

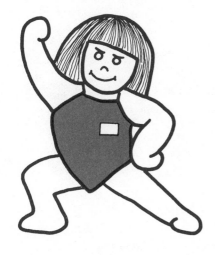

With the increase in swimming schools, there has been a corresponding proliferation of special swimming classes for mothers and children or for nursery school children, all of which have the common goal of encouraging physical development.

The swimming classes for nursery school children in a certain district of Tokyo are unique in that more than half of the children actually learn to swim, rather than just becoming accustomed to the water. Also, the district itself organizes the program and provides the instruction. All together, there are five nursery schools which participate. The following is a description of the last meeting of the five-class program.

Warm-ups

1. Do warm-up calisthenics in a circle around the edge of the pool.

2. March: Climb in the water and walk in a circle around the inside edge of the pool, paddling with the arms.

3. Seesaw: Face and hold hands in pairs. At the whistle, one partner crouches under water to the count of 3, then stands while the other crouches.

4. Underwater somersault: Put arms around the knees and do somersaults.

5. Bead hunt: Different-colored beads are scattered in the pool. At the signal "Red," the children dunk under water to find red beads, and so on.

"Don't be afraid, Mama!"

6. Fishing: Divide into three groups. One at a time, each child approaches an instructor. Two m (2 yards) away, the child puts his face into the water and swims down between the instructor's legs. Three m (3 yards) behind the instructor, there is a weighted toy fish on the bottom of the pool. The child picks it up and stands. The instructor may help some children through his legs.

7. Kickboard relay: Holding a kickboard in front, the children swim around the instructors and return to their team. The instructors stand in the middle of the pool about 4 m (4 yards) from the children.

8. Jumping in feetfirst: There are many different ways to jump into the pool: body erect, body bent slightly forward, knees held to chest, and so on.

9. Crawl: The children had already learned the basic idea of the crawl in a previous class. Today, their formal swimming practice began by gradually introducing them to the headfirst dive. First the instructors laid them face down on benches, tilted the benches up, and slipped them headfirst into the water. Each child would swim across the pool and return to the end of his line. Next time around, the instructors sat them in little chairs and had them dive from that position. Finally, they had the children dive from a standing position, pushing off with one foot.

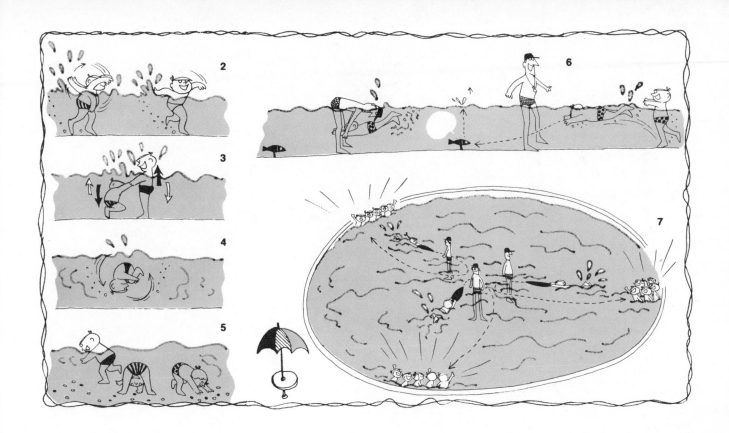

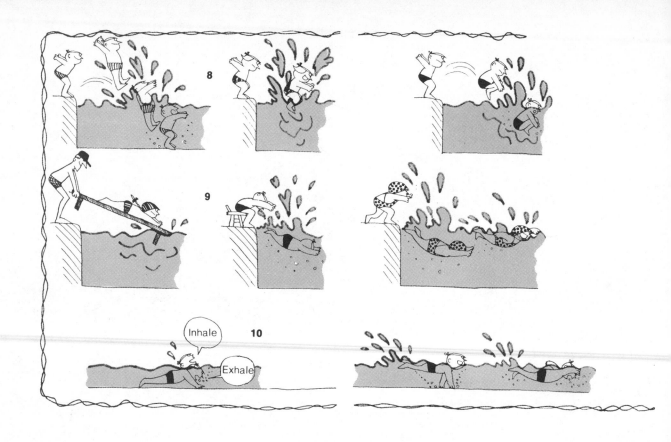

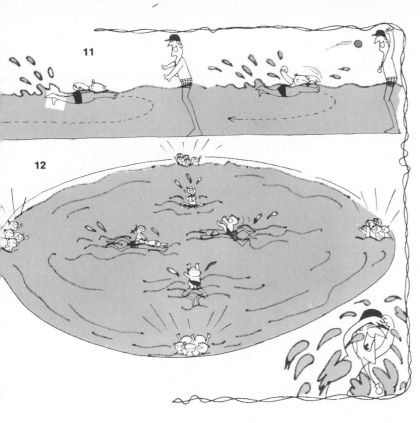

Meanwhile, an individual review session was given in a small vinyl pool beside the children's pool to those who still had not gained the knack of the breathing technique (**10**). In this shallow 30-cm (12-inch) pool, the children could keep their hands on the bottom, flutter-kick their legs, and practice the timing for inhaling and exhaling. As soon as a child could do this, he joined the others for diving and swimming.

11. Ball throwing: The instructor stands in the middle of the pool and the children swim to him one by one with a ball. They hand the ball to him and swim back. Next time, they can try to hit him with the ball before swimming back.

12. Boy on a dolphin: The instructors do the breaststroke back and forth in the pool with one child at a time riding on their backs. Some children can stay on all the way, some slip off and hold on by the instructor's neck, and others fall off completely. The children always enjoy this.

13. Finally, the children form a circle around the inside edge of the pool, with the instructors in the middle. The children all bow and say, "Thank you for teaching us," and then splash the instructors and one another.

After the children had showered and changed, they were presented with little badges. They left happily chattering with their mothers.

Chapter 49. Fitness for Students

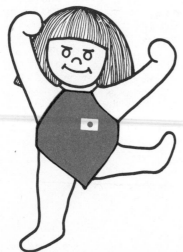

Beginning in September of each year, the physical education council of a certain city holds physical fitness clinics for students who are preparing for junior high school entrance exams, a very stressful event for Japanese youngsters. This clinic has gained such a good reputation that the once-a-week classes have been increased to accommodate the large number of participants. Classes are held every day of the week except Sunday, which is always citizen's sports day, and Monday, the sports center's regular holiday.

The basic idea of the clinic is that a child can best prepare for entrance exams by developing a healthy balance between body and mind. The clinic is coordinated with another special class for mothers whose children are preparing for exams.

There is no emphasis on one particular sport or another, and during rest periods, short talks are given on such topics as eating, studying, and sleeping habits. The aims of the clinic are to instill through physical exercise the ideal of "study hard, play hard," and to strengthen the will and capacity to study.

This chapter will describe a session which focused on exercises using the bamboo fencing sticks of kendo.

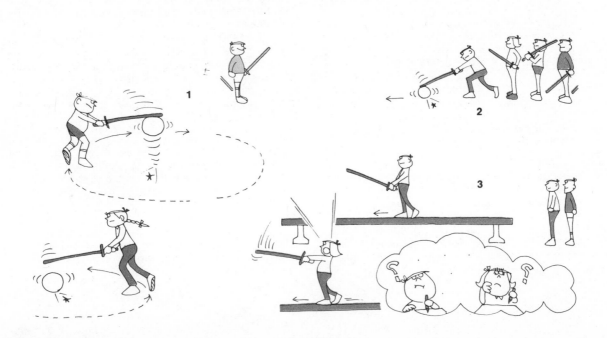

Warm-ups

1. Stick and ball: Each participant lightly bounces a gym ball with the tip of a fencing stick as he walks around it clockwise, then counterclockwise.

2. Ball relay: The class divides into five teams of ten each. These subdivide further into two halves facing each other over a distance. One by one, the contestants race over the distance with the ball, bouncing and controlling it with the kendo stick. The ball must not be allowed to get away from the stick.

3. Horizontal-bar kendo: Low horizontal bars are placed lengthwise in front of each team. The first time, the contestants slide along the bar with the stick in an "on guard" position. If a contestant falls, he or she must start over. The second time, the contestants slide along the bar while striking in the air with the stick and calling out, *"O-men!"* (touché) with each stroke.

4. Rest: During the short break, the participants practice writing Chinese characters.

Kendo practice

5. Touché: The participants stand sideways in a circle around the gym pointing their sticks, held in one hand at shoulder level, toward the center. One by one, the participants go around the circle striking the outstretched sticks with a strong overhead blow, each time calling out, *"O-men!"* When each has finished the circle, he takes his place with outstretched sword. Each person goes around twice.

6. Swift attack: The group divides into four sections, which one by one face off with the instructor. When he advances a step, they retreat a step. When he retreats, they advance. When he leaves an opening for such strokes as a mask stroke or body stroke, they respond accordingly, at the same time calling out vigorously the name of the stroke.

7. Attack practice: The instructor puts on full protective gear, and takes on the students one at a time. He shows one opening to each student, who responds with one swift stroke.

8. Ball striking: The group divides into five. One at a time, the students charge the teacher, who tosses out a rubber ball. Each student gets one downward stroke at it, yelling, *"O-men!"* at the same time.

9. Practice using protective equipment: The students take turns putting on the kendo protective gear, fencing in pairs for 3 minutes apiece.

Cooling down

10. "Scissors, paper, and stone" piggyback: The students play "scissors, paper, and stone" in pairs, and the loser carries the winner piggyback for 5 steps. They play again, and again loser carries winner 5 steps. In this way, they proceed around the gym twice.

11. Formal kneeling: Everyone kneels for 5 minutes in formal fashion, with buttocks resting on heels. The instructor lectures on proper posture and breathing.

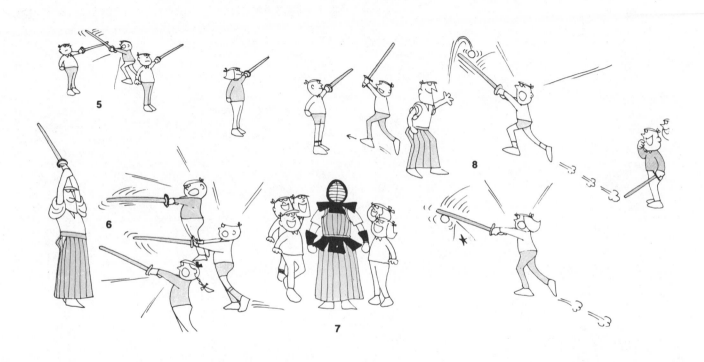

PART VI. FITNESS FOR SENIORS

Chapter 50. Exercise for Older People

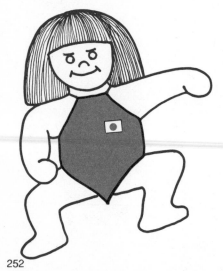

Mr. Toki is sixty-six, a retired professor who now lectures twice a week and spends the rest of his time reading, writing, working in the garden, and playing with his grandchildren. Despite the comforts of retirement, however, Mr. Toki suffers from failing legs and back. The simplest of garden tasks leaves him short of breath. His doctor's diagnosis was lack of exercise.

Mr. Toki was disturbed to hear this. What can an aging, unathletic scholar do for exercise, a scholar who all his life has believed in the superiority of mind over body? Walking, of course, is exercise, but Mr. Toki couldn't walk faster than a stroll.

The doctor told him about a physical fitness program that Europeans have developed for those over sixty. Under this program, the elderly exercise 30 minutes a day, even if they have to do it while lying in bed. This keeps them active and healthy, and helps them to enjoy life to the fullest. The doctor prescribed a weekly exercise plan with a different schedule for each day.

Monday

1. Ruler walking: Either indoors or outdoors, set a 30-cm (12-inch) ruler in front of you on the floor, and step from one end to the other. When your feet are together, crouch down, pick the ruler up from behind, and place it in front. Stand up and step again to the end of the ruler. Walk and crouch in this fashion for 5 minutes. As your legs become stronger, you may take a longer stride, eventually hopping the distance instead of stepping it, perhaps using a 60- or 90-cm (2- or 3-foot) stick.

2. Arm swinging: Stand with legs apart and a ruler in one hand. Pass the ruler to the other hand with a small swinging motion, then back to the original hand. As you pass it a third time, swing the arm that receives the ruler in an upward circle over the head and back down on the other side. The pattern of swings is small-small-large, small-small-large, and so on. Do this for 1 minute.

3. Ruler toss: Throw the ruler lightly into the air and catch it. Throw and catch it again, keeping a rhythm. Don't let it turn over in the air, or it will be difficult to catch. When you are ready, you may want to try a heavier object such as a book.

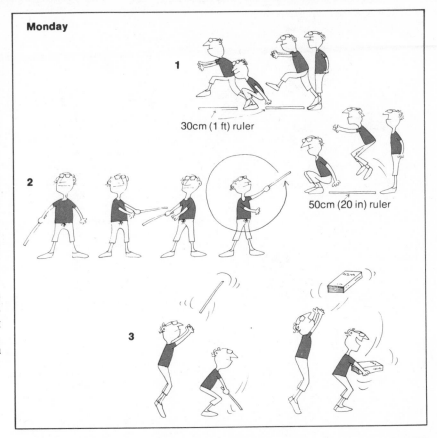

Monday

30cm (1 ft) ruler

50cm (20 in) ruler

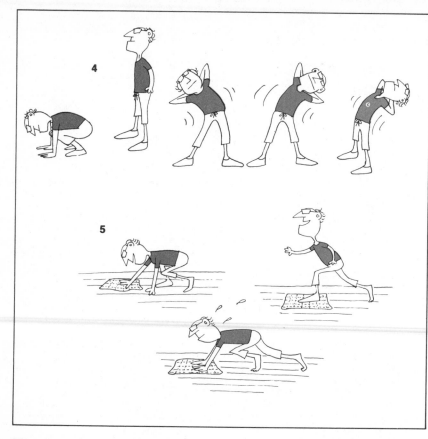

4. Stretching: Stand with legs apart. Bend knees, touch palms to the floor, and stand up. Do this 5 to 10 times. Then, with hands clasped behind neck, bend at the waist to the left, right, and backward. Do this 3 to 5 times.

5. Floor wiping: With a dry cloth, clean the floor of the kitchen, the hall, or some other uncarpeted part of the house. Do not kneel. Variations include riding the cloth with one foot and pushing with the other, and deck-cleaning, using both hands.

Tuesday

6. Tire jumping I: Bounce lightly on a discarded tire for 1 minute. When you have gained some confidence, you may try jumping higher, or changing direction while you jump.

7. Tire jumping II: Repeat the above for 1 minute, bringing legs together when you jump and spreading them when landing. Continue rhythmically.

8. Figure-eight tire rolling: Roll the tire in different-shaped figure eights—long narrow ones and short fat ones. See how many you can do in 3 minutes. Be sure to stay close behind the tire.

9. Knee stretching and back massage: Stand with legs as far apart as possible and hands on knees. Bend one knee and let yourself down, stretching the other knee well. Do this 5 times both left and right. With feet together and knees and upper torso bent slightly, pound from lower back down to calf muscles.

Tuesday

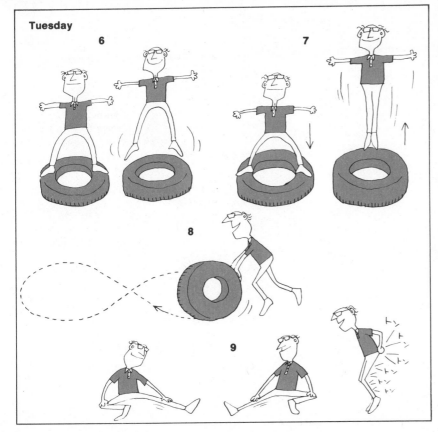

6   7

8

9

Wednesday

10. Skiing in place: Stand as if you were skiing on a flat surface, with feet together, knees and elbows flexed, and upper torso leaning slightly forward. That position being count 1, on count 2 swing elbows strongly backward, on 3 swing arms forward, at the same time straightening legs, and on 4 swing them back and bend knees. Do this 10 times.

11. Horizontal figure eights: Spread legs wide to the right and left and stretch both arms in front, wrists bent up so that the palms face forward. As you sway from foot to foot, describe horizontal figure eights with hands.

12. Circling in a push-up position: In a push-up position, move clockwise or counterclockwise in a circle which has hands at the center. You may spread legs slightly if necessary. Do 1 revolution.

13. Forward and reverse arm swinging: First warm up by gently rotating shoulders. Then swing both arms forward over head and back down in a large circle. At the top of the circle, clap hands. Repeat in the reverse direction. Do this 10 times in each direction.

Thursday

14. Golf swings: Thirty times, with or without a club.

15. Sidestepping: Lay three golf clubs 60 cm (2 feet) apart on the floor and step sideways back and forth over them for 3 minutes.

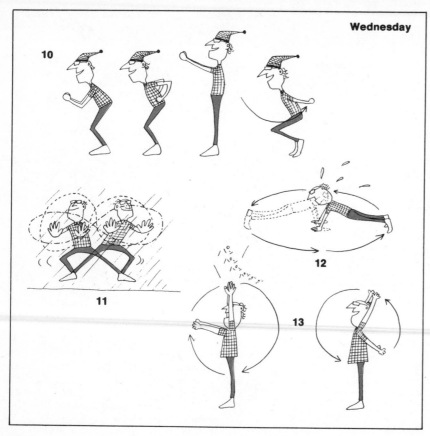

Wedneday

10

11

12

13

16. Putting practice: Using one golf ball, practice putting at a distance of 3 m (3 yards). Make 20 holes, no matter how many putts it takes for each hole.

Friday

17. Walk a 1-km (half-mile) course in 30 minutes. The second time out, do it in 25 minutes; the third time, in 22 minutes; and the fourth time, in 20 minutes. Exercise arms and shoulders while walking. If you like, you may run slowly part of the way.

Saturday

18. Sword cuts with a bamboo stick: Do 50 cuts. Use light footwork.

19. Sword thrusts with bamboo stick: Do 50 thrusts.

20. Abdominal breathing: Expand stomach only as you inhale deeply. Also try expanding both chest and stomach. Do this 10 times.

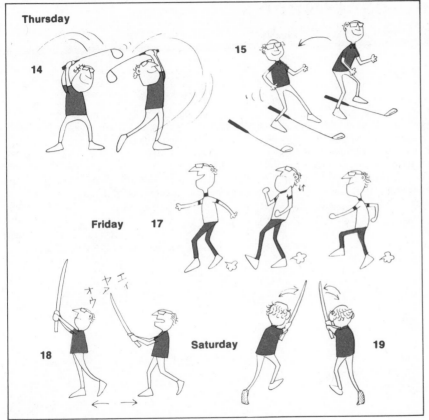

Thursday

14

15

Friday 17

18

Saturday 19

Sunday

Sunday is for rest. If your muscles are stiff, have someone give you a massage.

One month after beginning his exercise program, Mr. Toki happened to meet his doctor on the street and was happy to report that his legs and back no longer gave him trouble. He now owned running shoes and helped his wife with the housecleaning. The doctor remarked that Mr. Toki looked much healthier than he had a month earlier. Mr. Toki proudly responded that recently several of his students had told him he looked younger. "I'm sorry now that I didn't start exercising thirty years ago," he said.

After they had parted, the doctor remembered that he had been neglecting his own exercise program, and was inspired by Mr. Toki's example to return to it with renewed vigor.

Chapter 51. Fitness for Older Women

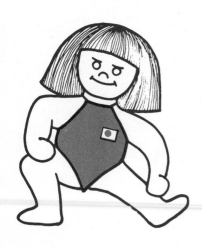

Japanese women in their forties and fifties are a group apart in modern Japan. Their childhood was dominated and distorted by the sufferings of war and deprivation. It is partly for this reason that many of them feel somehow unable to participate in the sports classes and physical fitness clinics for mothers which are proliferating. The pace in such classes is too fast, and spiritually these women feel a discontinuity between themselves and the younger generation. They experience a sense of alienation from much that is going on around them.

While certainly not all women of this generation customarily wear the traditional kimono, many of them do, and it is understandable that they feel inhibited from making a quick and easy adjustment to Western clothing, to say nothing of the rambunctiousness of modern sports.

This chapter will suggest exercises suitable to the life-style of women who wear traditional clothing, and to many other older women as well.

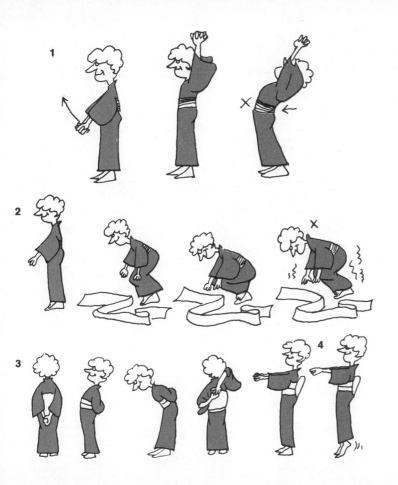

When dressing

1. Clasp hands and raise arms in front until palms are facing ceiling *without arching back.*

2. Pick up obi (a cloth belt for the kimono) or a modern belt with one foot placed on top of the other.

3. Clasp hands behind back and raise them together to touch shoulder blades. If you can't reach this high the first day, try to get a little higher the next. Watch your progress each day. It is all right to bend forward, but even better to arch your back slightly in doing this task. A similar exercise is to touch fingers behind back by stretching right arm over right shoulder, and left arm up from below.

4. Stand erect with feet together, arms extended in front and eyes closed. Rise on tiptoe and keep balance to the count of 8. Remember that one sign of aging is a decrease in the ability to keep one's balance.

Do the above four tests every day as a way of keeping tabs on your physical condition—a kind of physical fitness barometer.

259

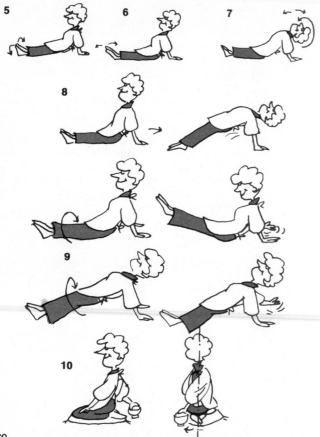

When taking a break

Two or three times a day, most women take a short break from their chores. During this time, sit on the tatami (straw-mat) floor with feet extended and do the following exercises.

5. Slowly, but firmly, rotate ankles.

6. Stretch toes as far forward as possible.

7. With arms extended back for support, slowly rotate neck in large circles. Also stretch neck forward and back.

8. In the same position, raise torso to make a straight line, and hold it to the count of 5. This will require exerting strength throughout whole body. Do it once each time you take a break.

9. Supported by your arms, lift and rotate legs. First make small circles, then gradually larger ones. If you do this exercise faithfully, the day will come when you can remove the support of one of your arms.

10. After drinking a cup of tea in the customary kneeling position, place the emptied cup behind you with one hand. At first, you should be able to place it at least directly behind you. Later, when greater flexibility develops, or if you lose some weight, you should be able to place it far on the other side. That is, if you are using your right hand, you should be able to place the cup well over to the left.

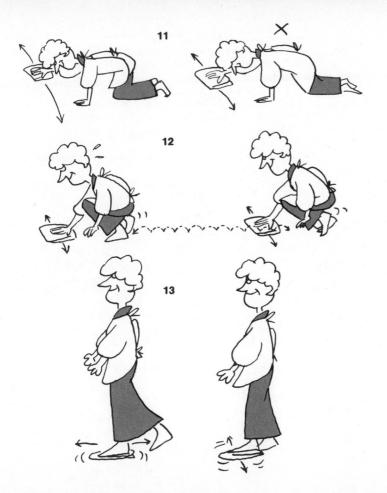

When dusting the floor

Though on the average there is less floor space in individual dwellings than there once was, most housewives dust one floor or another almost every day.

11. When kneeling to dust, use large arm motions and keep stomach contracted.

12. When stooping, use small, quick hand motions, and move along with small steps. This will improve stamina. Those who are overweight will find that they get out of breath fairly soon in this position, but they should not give up. With determination, things will get better.

13. Dusting with one foot on the dustcloth is good exercise for the legs.

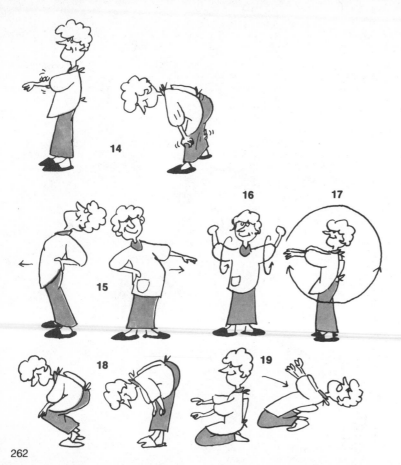

When taking a momentary breather

There are moments when, involved in one chore or another, one stops for a brief rest, perhaps to massage shoulders if they are sore or to rotate the neck if it feels stiff. Such moments are almost below the level of consciousness. Try to make the following exercises part of your repertoire of unconscious habits.

14. Learn the important *tsubo* (pressure points) of *shiatsu* (finger massage), and apply pressure to some of them, particularly the outer concave spots just below the knees and elbows.

15. Arch back with hands at lower back. Think of this exercise as pushing thighs forward or to the sides.

You will be surprised at the extent to which your physical condition will improve if you can make these exercises an unconscious part of your habitual routine. The best proof of this will be when you find that you can do with ease something that you did with difficulty before.

Even if you do wear the traditional and somewhat confining kimono, when you dress in the morning or undress for a bath or for bed, use larger, more vigorous motions. Rotate your shoulders (**16**), rotate your arms (**17**), and bend forward with hands on knees (**18**). Before you go to sleep, kneel on your bed and bend over backward, as in yoga (**19**).

Chapter 52. Fitness Activities for Senior Citizens

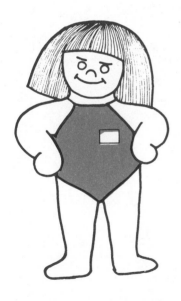

In a certain Japanese industrial city, every citizen upon reaching sixty-five is presented with a "longevity memorandum book," given free-admission privileges to various public events, and granted other special benefits. As part of the medical welfare system, a sound body physical fitness program is also offered, which among other things sponsors folk-singing and folk-dancing classes and early-morning walk groups. Out of this program there also emerged a group for sports lovers, affectionately called the Sparrow Sports Club after the Japanese proverb which says that even into old age, sparrows never forget how to flutter and dance. This club meets two mornings a month at the city's sports center. More than twenty members participate.

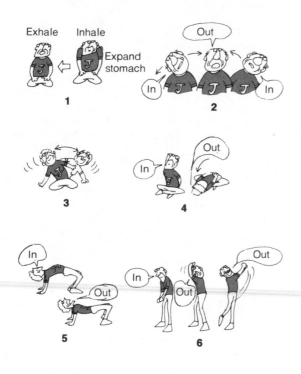

Warm-ups (with emphasis on breathing)

1. Shoulder lifts (10 times): Sit with back erect in formal kneeling position, with the instep of the left foot resting on the arch of the right. As you inhale, raise shoulders and expand stomach (not chest). As you exhale, let shoulders down naturally.

2. Neck stretching (10 times left and right): Inhale while stretching, and exhale while returning to normal position.

3. Side bends (10 times left and right): Relax shoulders and swing to the sides like an upside-down pendulum.

4. Forward bending (10 times): Sit cross-legged and with back erect as in Zen meditation. Clasp hands behind back. Exhale as you bend forward, and inhale as you return.

5. Back arching (10 times): In a four-legged position facing *upward,* arch back and chest and lift stomach as you inhale; let them down as you exhale.

6. Body twisting (10 times): Stand as if holding a golf club and inhale. Exhale slowly as you make the backswing, and as you make the shot, exhale strongly.

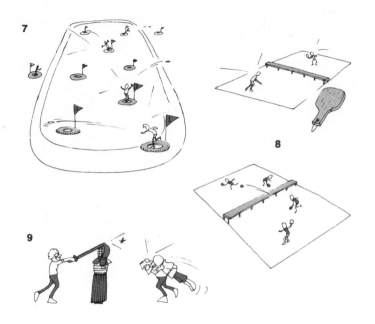

7

8

9

Frisbee golf

7. Play "golf," using nine discarded tires for holes and Frisbees for balls. The tires should be an average of 75 m (80 yards) apart, par for the course being 36. This is an economical and enjoyable way to get the leg exercise which is so important in slowing the process of aging. Before discovering this game, the Sparrow Sports Club had tried to keep up its early morning walks. That effort failed because the activity of walking was not interesting enough in itself and because it was difficult to find a pace which satisfied all. The shift to games brought a new increase in interest and participation.

Beach bat

8. Use wooden paddles and a tennis ball, a Ping-Pong ball, or a badminton bird. Play on a makeshift court 3 m (3 yards) wide and 10 m (11 yards) long, with benches placed across the middle for a net. Limit play to 20 minutes so that no one gets overexerted.

Cooling down

9. After putting the above equipment away, practice kendo (bamboo fencing) or judo against a dummy.

As the men walk home in twos and threes in their training suits, they are greeted by students and office workers on the way to school and the office. This lifts their spirits and gives them a sense of belonging to the workaday world.

Chapter 53. A Senior Citizens' Sports Festival

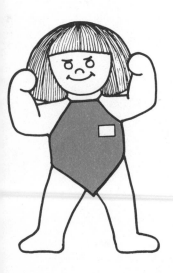

Because of the growing membership and enthusiasm of its senior citizen sports club, folk-singing club, and early-morning walk club, a certain Japanese town decided to establish an annual senior citizens' sports festival. Anyone over sixty was eligible, and the mayor and other public figures participated, lending an air of significance to the event. Children and grandchildren came out to support their family's representatives, and all in all, it was a festive, fun-filled half day.

In this town, it had become something of a custom to celebrate a senior citizen's sixtieth birthday with the presentation of a new training suit or running shoes, so all the participants were well equipped for the festival. Also, on the day of the festival itself, each participant was given a free pair of sports *tabi*, a kind of traditional footwear which is a cross between shoes and socks.

The festival was organized jointly by the committees on welfare and physical education, but much of the actual preparation was carried out by the Boy Scouts, Girl Scouts, and teenage sports groups. The following is a description of the day's events.

Processional

To thunderous applause and the music of a recorded march, about one hundred participants paraded into the athletic grounds. As they marched, they waved and held up imitation roses which had been passed out by the Girl Scouts. There was a speech by the chairman of the organizing committee, and another by the mayor, in behalf of the participants.

Warm-up exercises

1. For warm-ups, the participants formed two concentric circles, and for 10 minutes danced to various well-known folk songs.

Bowling

2. From a distance of 7 m (8 yards), participants tried to knock over a pin with a dodge ball or volleyball. Anyone able to do this 3 times won a prize.

Haiku relay

3. This is something which perhaps only Japanese can do, because of the tradition of linked poetry. Instead of carrying a baton, the competitors carry a writing brush. The first on each team runs to a large piece of paper attached to a wall and writes the first line of a poem. He then runs back and passes the brush to a teammate, who runs up and improvises the next line, and so on. This event is especially popular because it exercises both the mind and body. For each team there should be a reader who stands near the sheets of paper and reads each line aloud to the spectators after it has been written.

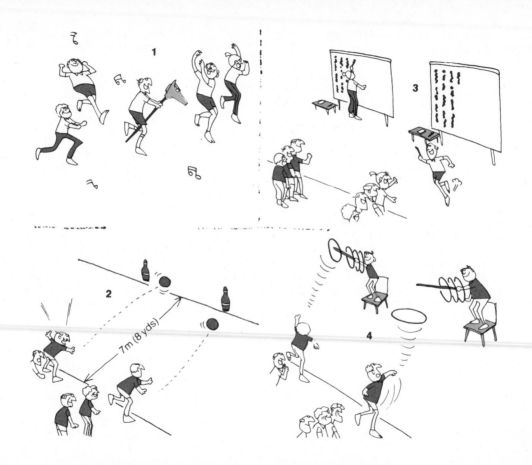

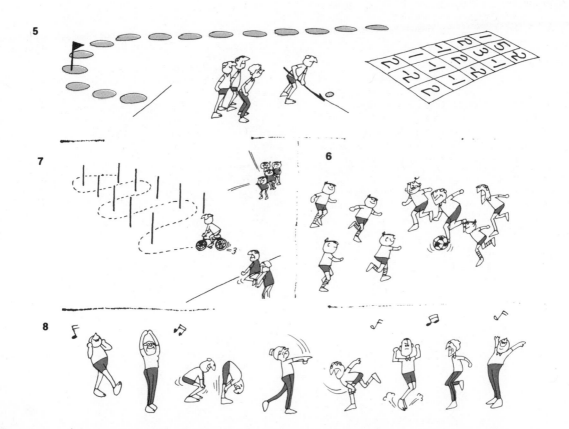

Ringtoss relay

4. Each participant in turn tosses two rings apiece to a teenager who stands at a distance on a chair or platform and tries to catch the rings with a pole. The team which makes the most ringers wins.

Shuttleboard backgammon

5. A rectangular board is laid out and numbered as in drawing, including some minus figures. Using a sponge mop, the participants on each team alternately push a hockey puck into the rectangle, and advance or return their flag along a course according to the number of the square in which the puck lands. The first flag to reach the end of the course wins.

Various exhibitions

6. Exhibitions are given of various Japanese martial arts such as *aikidō*, *kendo*, and *judo*. Also, a short soccer match is held between those over sixty and those under sixteen.

Zigzag cycling race

7. Participants ride a 14-inch child's bicycle over a zigzag course laid out with five pairs of poles set at 3-m (3-yard) intervals. An old-timer should feel a half century younger when riding his grandchild's bicycle.

The town's physical fitness song

8. To promote wider interest and participation in exercise and sports, a town physical fitness song had been selected, and a standard series of exercises was designed to go along with the first three verses. Everyone from grandchildren on up knew it and could join in.

Closing ceremony

Medallions were passed out to all the participants, and "keys to health" were awarded to ten whose performance was particularly distinguished. It was a fun-filled and healthy two hours for both participants and spectators.

Chapter 54. Outdoor Recreation Areas

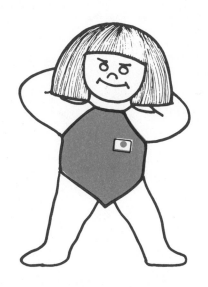

There has been active debate recently over the need for more athletic facilities. This recognition of the importance of physical exercise to the health of our society is belated, but welcome nonetheless. However, more than half of the facilities under consideration are for schools, and not open to the general public. The other half, provided of necessity by local governments, is largely for sports such as baseball and tennis, which serve only a small part of the population. The original need has gone largely unfilled.

There are other and more desirable solutions than those we have seen thus far.

For example, plans for new apartment complexes should provide for a running track, a playground for children, a swimming pool, a sauna, and other basic facilities. After work a person should be able to exercise and maintain his fitness and health on the grounds of his own home, rather than depending on commercial sports facilities.

At this point, however, one can only wish. In the meantime, there are many ways to improve the available spaces and the ways in which they are used. Let us look at some of them in this chapter.

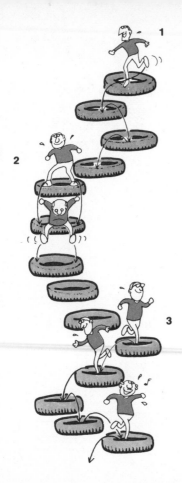

For 30 x 20m
(35 x 25 yd) area

On the outer edge of the area used, set a number of discarded tires at either regular or irregular intervals.

1. Run across the tops of the tires. If the distances between them are large, jump; if small, run quickly without missing a step. This will strengthen your ankles, improve your balance, and test your agility.

2. With legs spread the width of the tires, jump from one to the next, seeing how many you can jump without stopping. This will provide both a challenge and a record of stamina improvement.

3. Set the tires in a zigzag course and run in the center of them. It will be even more of a challenge if you step into the tires on the right with your left foot and into the tires on the left with your right foot.

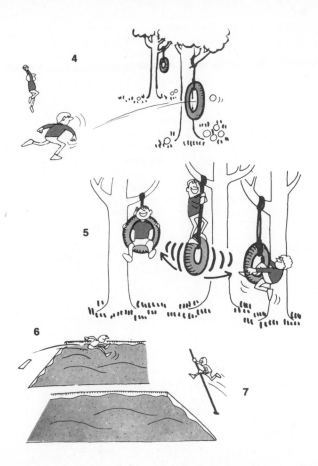

Suspend tires at the outer edge of the area.

4. If the tire is suspended near a wall, it can be used for pitching practice.

5. Children can use the suspended tires as swings. Or they can perhaps swing from one to the next like Tarzan.

Put a sandbox in the center.

6. Set a takeoff plank into the ground, and calibrate the side of the box to measure standing and running broad jumps.

7. Set another plank into the ground on the other side of the box for jumping with a pole. Provide poles of various lengths and thicknesses.

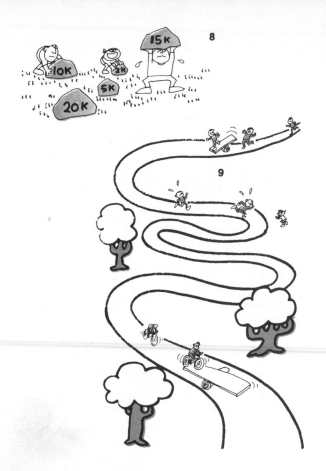

8. Make a collection of rocks and paint its weight on each. Try your hand at weight lifting.

9. Lay out a zigzag or wavelike course 1 m (1 yard) wide for running or bicycling. At several points along the way, place an obstacle such as a strong board set across a small log.

The cost for such facilities is minimal, less than any one piece of standard playground equipment, and the uses to which they can be put are many. Until now, vacant spaces have usually been left vacant and unused, or they have been used for baseball. It is important that the space not be co-opted by a special-interest group for one particular sport or another. It is also important that there be instructions and cautions posted so that first-time users will be able to become involved in activities right away. The more users the better, because they will support the building of new facilities in the future.

In this chapter, I have suggested ways to use a relatively small area. If your neighborhood has a larger area, you can probably think of many other innovative ways to put it to good use.

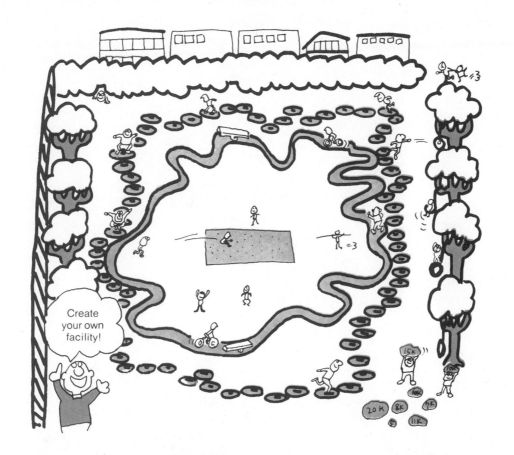

Chapter 55. An Exercise Retreat for Mothers and Children

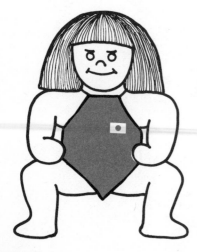

Another partial solution to the urgent need for exercise facilities in crowded urban areas is for municipal governments to purchase land in nearby rural sectors and to build there for the use of their citizens. A certain Japanese city plagued by pollution and other urban hazards did just that. Five years ago it purchased a half acre of land and constructed a dormitory which could sleep seventy persons, two in each room.

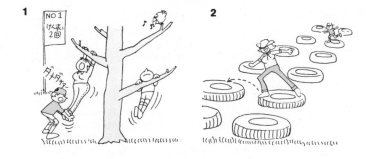

Let us look in this chapter at the three-day schedule of an exercise retreat which was held there for mothers and their fifth- and sixth-grade children.

Day 1

Two buses arrived in the early afternoon. Room assignments were made and everyone immediately changed clothes, wearing the straw sandals which had been provided at the dormitory. Ten minutes by foot from the dormitory is a large pasture which covers both sides of a hill. A 4-km (2½-mile) course, equipped with fifteen exercise positions, is laid out in this pasture. For two hours the members of the group enjoyed themselves along this course.

1. Chin-ups: An appropriate tree had been designated for chin-ups. Everyone was supposed to do 2, though many of the mothers couldn't do even one. Those who had difficulty were given a boost by their children.

2. Tire hopping: Tires were lined up in two staggered rows. Participants progressed down them 3 times by jumping back and forth from one row to the other.

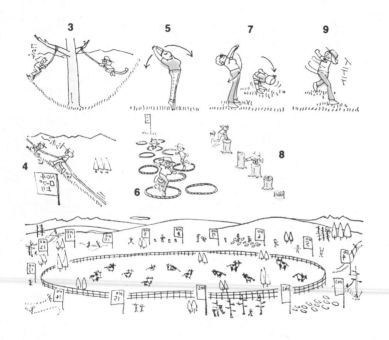

3. Tarzan: Ropes had been hung from branches of a tree which grew in a dip in the land. Participants would take the rope on one side of the dip and swing to the other. Only five of the mothers dared to challenge this obstacle, but all five were successful and were duly applauded.

4. Rope climbing: Ten-m (11-yard) ropes were attached to the top of a rather steep slope so that participants could pull themselves up.

5. Stretching and twisting: Each person breathes deeply, stretching on tiptoe with hands over head, and twists body twice to right and left.

6. Ring hopping: Large rope rings were laid out over a level area, and participants hopped on one leg from one ring to the next. This activity made the mothers feel that they had become children again.

7. Forward bending: Participants bend forward from the waist, bounce back up, and stretch arms over head 3 times.

8. Stump leaping: Participants choose a row of stumps which is best for their height, and vault over them as in leapfrog.

9. Torso twisting: Place one foot forward and twist torso to left and right with arms extended.

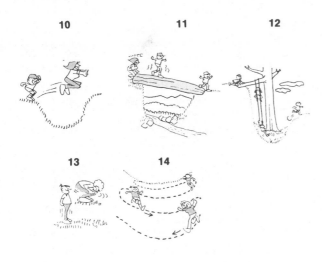

11. Log crossing: Two m (2 yards) beneath a log, a little brook flowed. It was surprising how many were frightened of falling in.

12. Pole sliding: Two climbing poles were hanging from a tree branch which could be approached from a nearby bank. Participants slide down, jumping the last meter (yard).

13. Knee bends: Bend at knees as far as possible without letting heels leave ground.

14. Zigzag running: Participants run zigzag down the gently sloped ditch.

15. Arm swinging: Participants swing arms in large circles forward, then backward, 3 times each.

Everyone left the pasture at the gate where they had entered. They were tired, and some had sore feet from the straw sandals, but everybody felt happy and healthy. When they got back, some soaked their feet in the stream flowing in front of the dormitory. Others went directly to the large bath. For supper they were served deep-fat-fried tempura, including that made with various locally grown vegetables.

10. Broad jump: Near the top of the hill there was a ditch. Each person jumps back and forth over a section which is suitably wide. This also is the best place to rest, so everyone lies in the grass and enjoys the sun and breeze. In this open environment, contrasting so sharply with the crowded city, the children have already begun to make new friends, even though they are from different schools.

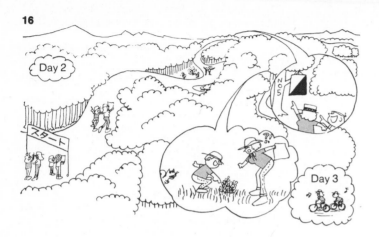

16

edible plants, much to their dismay. All in all, however, the morning was a great success.

In the afternoon the children divided into two groups, one for hiking around a nearby lake and the other for mountain climbing. The mothers stayed behind and made preparations for an outdoor barbecue.

Day 3

From 9:00 to 11:00, everyone went cycling. Their route was quite a change from the restricted urban areas where the children usually bicycled. There also were a number of places along the route which were so steep that many had to get off their bikes and walk.

This short retreat in the midst of nature, away from the dehumanizing forces of the city, was a wonderful experience for both parents and children. And, most important, it was an invigorating three days which hopefully instilled or rekindled in all the spirit of physical fitness and exercise. In high spirits, the happy party sang their way back to the city on board the buses.

Day 2

Before breakfast, everyone went for a walk. From 8:00 to 9:30 was free time for reading or drawing. Then, from 10:00 to 11:30, a Scandinavian orienteering meet was held (**16**). First, everyone was taught how to use a map and compass. Then they were sent off in parent-child pairs with the task of finding three kinds of edible plants, such as *fuki* (butterbur) or *obako* (plantain). Of the twenty spots to be located in the meet, there were five which nobody could find. There were also couples who brought back quite in-

Chapter 56. A Children's Ski Trip

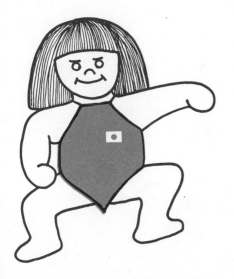

The most common form that physical activity takes during the cold winter months is, of course, skiing and skating, the so-called winter sports. These are commonly thought of as adult sports, but there is no reason why they can't be introduced to young children. In a major Japanese urban center, a winter sports outing for five- and six-year-olds has been held for the past five years at a retreat in the snow country up north. During the spring and summer these facilities are used for various school excursions, but in the fall and winter they are opened to the general public of the district. The retreat is quite popular, partly because of its hot-spring baths.

In this chapter, I will describe the activities of a three-day program organized in winter for first- and second-graders.

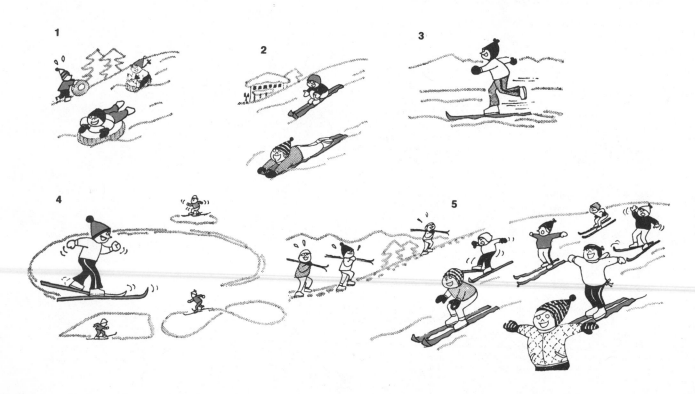

Day 1

Upon arrival about noon, rooms were assigned, and everyone hurried to change clothes and get outside. When the party had reassembled, it was divided into five teams of ten children each.

1. Tire sliding: Old tires were used for sliding down a gentle slope. Each team had five tires. On the first run, the children sat on their tires. When they reached the bottom, they would roll it back up the hill. If it got away, they would run after it, slipping and sliding. This gave the children a chance to get used to the slope and the snow. The second time, the children slid belly down. On the third run, a distance competition was held.

2. Ski sliding: Next, skis without harnesses or metal edges were distributed, and the children used them for sliding, either sitting or lying on their bellies.

3. One-footed skiing: The children were given one ski apiece to try without poles on a flat, well-packed surface. At first, they were instructed to walk on the skiless foot, then encouraged to propel themselves gradually with a kicking motion. After 15 minutes, they changed the ski to the other foot.

4. Making tracks: Next, the children were fitted with a second ski, and instructed to make big and small circles, figure eights, and squares. By this time, they were quite comfortable on the skis and could move with some speed.

5. The first run: Finally, the children were allowed to ski down a long, gentle slope, carrying their skis on their shoulders as they walked back up.

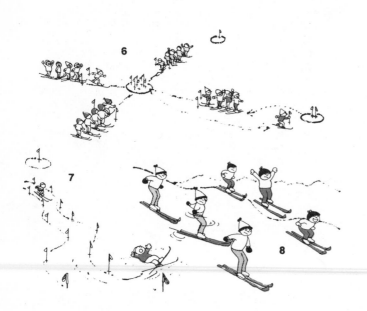

Day 2

6. Pole race: This time, teams competed as shown in the drawing. Ski poles were placed in a circle, and the child at the head of the line on each team would ski up to the circle, pull out a pole, and carry it as fast as he could to the far side. When he had done this, he would return to begin a line on the opposite side.

7. Mini-slalom: An easy slalom course is laid out with ski poles.

8. Downhill skiing: After the children had learned to turn without using poles and were relatively comfortable on skis, they began to ski in earnest. Still using the long, gentle slope, and carrying the skis back up after each run, they practiced various techniques such as crouching down or turning with light tail-jumps. An adult who has never skied before would be envious of the remarkable progress which children can make.

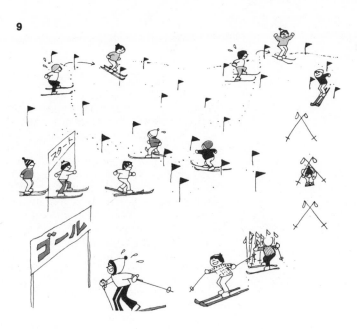

9

Day 3

Because this was the last day and there was a long bus ride home, the children could ski for only two hours in the morning. Using ski poles as markers, a course was laid out in such a way that all the skills acquired would be used—a kind of review test (**9**). At the starting line the ground was level, but from there on, without poles, the children had to climb, ski downhill, climb again, crouch low through a tunnel made of crossed poles, and then take poles for a final dash to the finish line. Each child went over the course three to five times.

On the first day of the outing, some of the children had difficulty adjusting to the unfamiliar surroundings, but by the time it came to leave, all were happy, and the bus trip home was lots of fun.

Chapter 57. Exercise Facilities at Work

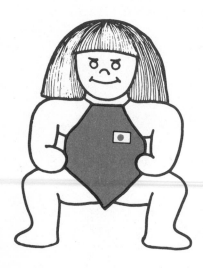

Mr. Hino was the health program manager in a factory which was built on a site covering 100,000 square meters (approximately 25 acres). For the company's five-hundred employees there were two tennis courts, one volleyball court, and an area where softball or other games could be played.

At lunchtime, all the play areas were usually filled immediately with about twice as many spectators along the sidelines as participants. In good weather, most of the women would walk about or lie in the grass and talk.

Mr. Hino considered submitting plans for a new gymnasium, but such a facility would necessarily be limited in the number of people it could accommodate at one time, and the costs were prohibitive. After much consideration, Mr. Hino came up with the following suggestions, which he presented before a meeting of those concerned with the problem:

Construction of a 350-m (380-yard) "beauty and health promenade" around the perimeter of the existing athletic field.

Construction of five to seven spots around the promenade fitted with appropriate exercise equipment.

Posting of instructions at each spot on how to use the equipment.

Mr. Hino's suggestions were approved unanimously, and steps were taken for their implementation. This chapter will describe each of the exercise spots placed along the promenade.

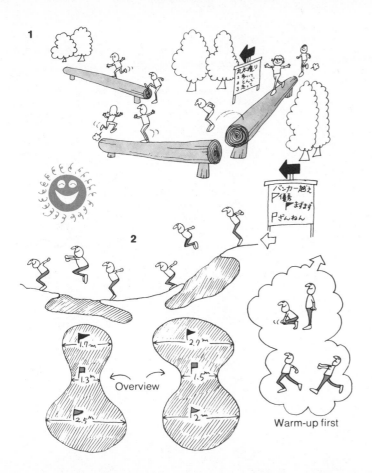

Overview

Warm-up first

1. Log walking: Logs of different thicknesses are installed at different heights, one or several at a slight incline. A sign suggests, in order of difficulty, three ways of crossing the logs: walking, hopping with feet together, and running. These logs can be used in a variety of ways, one of which, of course, is as a place to sit and talk. But more often, they encourage employees to be active and energetic.

2. Bunker jumping: Several sand bunkers in the shape of gourds are set into the natural configuration of the land. Employees who are not confident in the strength of their legs can start by jumping where the bunker is narrower, increasing the distance as they feel able. Of course, if one doesn't quite make the distance, he only lands in sand. It is wise to post a suggestion that employees do some warm-up exercises before jumping, especially deep knee bends and stretching of the Achilles tendon.

3. Parallel-bar strength tests: Two sets of parallel bars are installed, one low for arm-walking, the other high for chin-ups or monkey-swinging. Women can set their aim at covering half the distances.

4. Ball throwing: A softball-throwing range of 15 m (16 yards) is provided (a). For women, there is a volleyball throwing range, with a basketball hoop fixed 10 cm (4 inches) off the ground and 7 m (8 yards) from the throwing line (b).

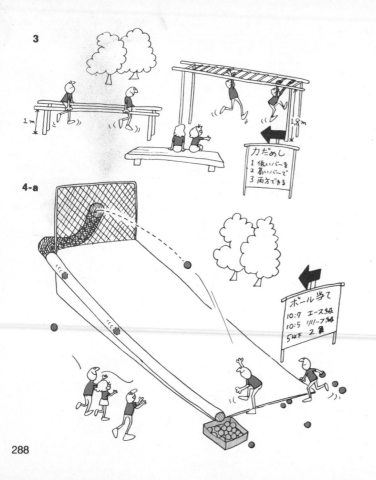

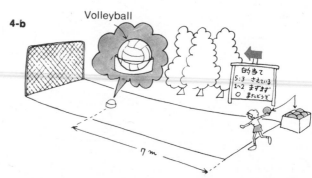

Volleyball

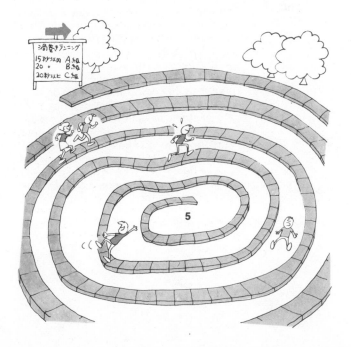

5. Whirlpool running course: There is a 100-m (110-yard) brick running course in the shape of a whirlpool.

6. Kickball: A soccer ball hangs from a tree limb with rope and a net. The response of a kicked ball will vary greatly depending on the length of the rope, but the suggested length is 2.5 m (8 feet), with the ball 5 cm (2 inches) above ground. A circle should be drawn on the ground (or imagined) with a center directly below the hanging ball and a radius of 1 m (1 yard). Anyone who without stepping out of the circle can kick the ball 5 times in succession is a "great kicker," and anyone who kicks it 3 times in succession has potential. Anyone who does less than this needs practice. It is, of course, possible to make the rope length adjustable. Mr. Hino, however, had the idea of using a 2-m (6-foot) rubber rope, which made the action of the ball more difficult to predict, and therefore more challenging.

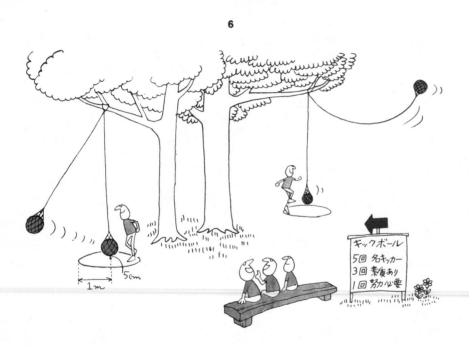

6

キックボール
5回 名キッカー
3回 素質あり
1回 努力必要

One month after the promenade had been completed, there were not many employees who could achieve perfect marks on all the tasks. But the course received a great deal of use during the lunch hour and breaks, a marked change from the time when most people stood idly about watching the active few. Many who had had no interest in physical exercise began to use the new facility. There were also some enthusiastic employees who would come early just to go once around the course before work.

The great virtue of the "beauty and health promenade," and the reason why it is so successful with both management and workers, is its flexibility. It fills a variety of needs, and can be used or altered to respond to a variety of situations. All those who are seriously interested in employee health and fitness would do well to reconsider old attitudes toward sports and recreation facilities, even if only as a way to help employees follow up on physical fitness tests.

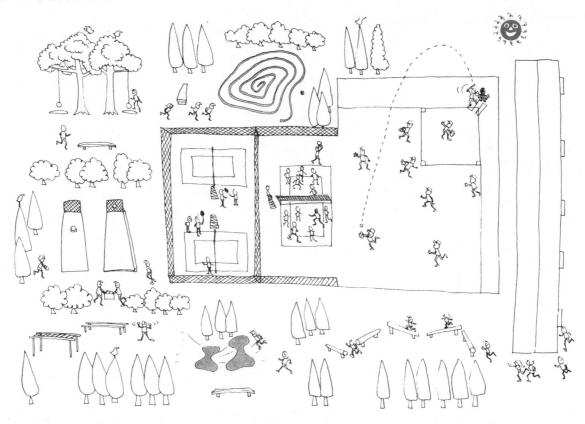

Chapter 58. Group Games at Work

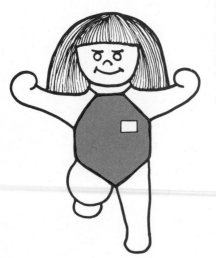

Five years ago, a manufacturing company on the island of Shikoku instituted a full-fledged physical fitness program for its three thousand employees. As an important part of this program, various outings and retreats were organized in groups of two hundred at different times of the year. Every year in the early summer an orienteering meet was held, and in the late summer, a great physical fitness festival. In the fall, smaller athletic meets were held. All this indicated the determination of the company to succeed in its physical fitness program, no small matter considering that the factory was on a round-the-clock production schedule.

In this chapter, I will introduce two of the group games which gained particular popularity among the employees before and after their shifts.

Handminton

This is a form of badminton developed in West Germany which uses hands in place of rackets. It provides a surprising amount of exercise, even when played with four on a side.

The court is 10 m (11 yards) long and 5 m (5 1/2 yards) wide, and the net is 1.8 m (2 yards) high. As in volleyball or ordinary badminton, there are 15 points to a game. If both sides are tied at 14 points apiece, one side must win by 2 points. If many people are waiting, 11-point games may be played.

The service area is behind the base line within 2 m of the right side of the court. The server gets only one chance for each point, and must serve underhanded. Once the shuttlecock enters the opposite court, the players may hit it up to 3 times in returning it. If the serving side wins a volley, it earns a point. If the receiving side wins a volley, it earns the right to serve, though not a point. In other words, the right to serve has to be earned first. Only then can a point be won. In this respect, the rules are similar to those of volleyball.

An experienced player hits the shuttlecock with his fingers, not with his palm, and he gives a snap of the wrist. Beginners should practice passing in a circle in order to observe how the shuttlecock behaves and to get a feel for hitting it with the fingers.

Ring tennis

Also called deck tennis, this game has been played for years on ocean liners. Instead of a ball, rubber rings are tossed back and forth over a net. As in handminton, it may be played with one, two, or more players on a side.

The server gets only one serve. The receiver must catch the ring with only one hand and return it within 3 seconds. He may not take more than 2 steps before throwing it. There is a 1-m neutral area on both sides of the net. If the ring falls into the opponent's neutral area, the thrower loses the point. The scoring is the same as in handminton.

The above two games were developed in West Germany as part of a movement to increase general participation in sports. I wholeheartedly applaud that movement and encourage those who are helping to spread it in Japan, both at home and at work.

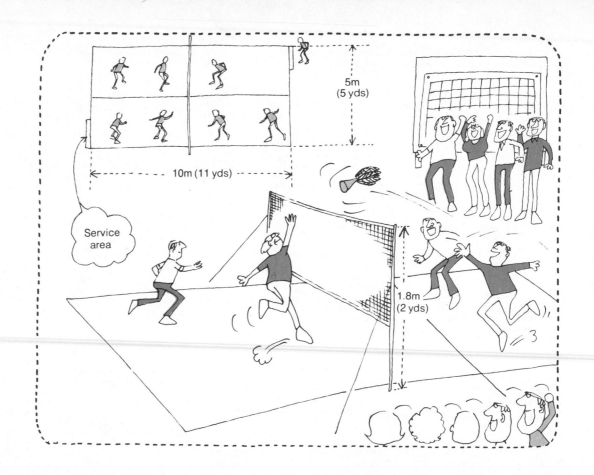

Service area

5m
(5 yds)

10m (11 yds)

1.8m
(2 yds)

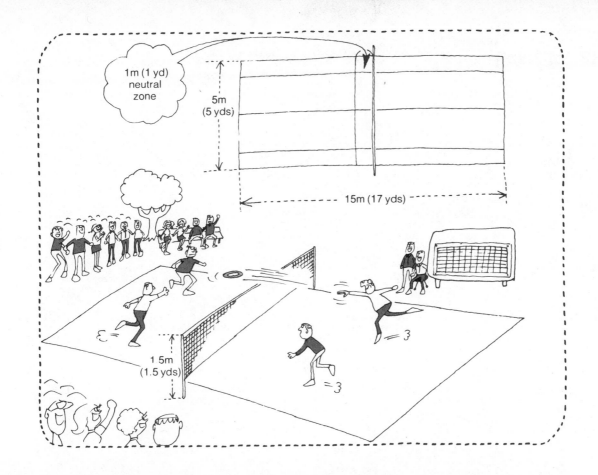

Chapter 59. A Training Retreat for Younger Employees

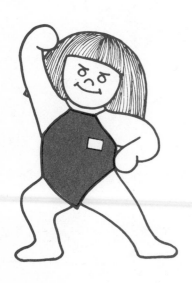

The day after they joined the company, eighty new employees of a certain Japanese organization began a four-day training retreat. These men were all recent graduates of either high school or college, and an important goal of the retreat was to instruct them in the internal operations and organization of the company. But even more important than this was the stress laid on the development in the men of a proper balance between body and spirit. The daily schedule was extremely demanding, because efficiency required that the new employees become professional almost overnight. They were thus expected to participate in all the retreat activities with great energy and concentration.

A special instructor was brought in to lecture on health management for men in their twenties. The following description of the first physical fitness workout he conducted is taken from the diary of one of the participants:

"All along, I had been struggling to keep up with the fast pace, countering my lack of confidence with a firm determination to succeed. But when it came to these sessions with the physical fitness instructor, I thought for sure that I would have no problems. After all, I had played volleyball in both high school and college and thought I was in good shape. I wasn't at all prepared for what happened. Here is the workout.

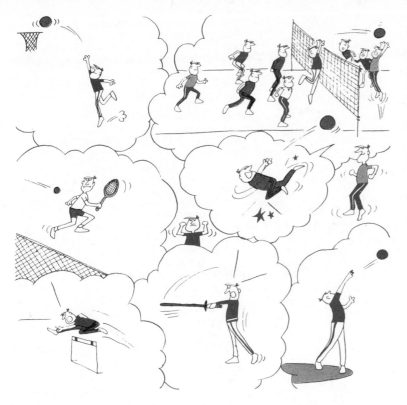

"First there were imitation exercises for 5 minutes. We were made to go through the motions of a number of different sports. We did tennis strokes and swimming strokes. We pretended to hurdle and to throw the shot-put, javelin, and hammer. And we did some volleyball returns. Finally, we did some quick kendo thrusts. Having done nothing before but ordinary calisthenics for warm-ups, I was totally surprised at all this. But I got good and warmed up.

"Then there were some physical fitness tests. We had to stand on one leg with the other wrapped behind at the knee, with our arms raised at the sides. We closed our eyes, slowly turned our heads to the right and then to the left, and repeated this on the other foot. This was more difficult than I imagined, and there wasn't one of us who could do it completely successfully. We had to laugh when we were told to be careful since there is a direct correlation between aging and one's sense of balance.

"Next, we had to kneel erect with our arms stretched at our sides for balance. Raising one leg behind, we bent down and touched our foreheads to the floor.

"Third, from a push-up position we had to thrust our legs in front through our arms so that we were facing up. I couldn't do it because my rear kept getting in the way.

Exercise Task Sheet

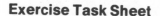

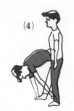

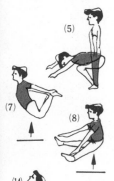

1) Walk 1 km (0.6 mile) in 10 minutes.
2) Run 1 km in 5 minutes.
3) Run up 5 flights of stairs without getting out of breath.
4) Touch toes 20 times.
5) Bend at knees and waist so that chest touches thighs 20 times.
6) Suck in stomach as hard as possible 5 times.
7) Jump and touch both heels behind with hands 5 times.
8) Jump and touch toes in front with hands 3 times.
9) Do standing broad jump to your height plus 30 cm (1 foot).
10) Jump to the sides, snapping legs together in air 10 times.
11) Jump right, left, back, and front with legs together for 60 seconds.
12) Balance on one leg with eyes closed for 40 seconds.
13) Jump rope 30 seconds and rest 1 minute; 1 minute and rest 1 minute; 1 minute and rest 30 seconds. Do this 3 times.
14) Bend backward and touch right heel with left hand and vice versa.
15) With hands clasped behind neck, bend at knees and waist to touch elbows to floor 3 times.
16) Do 20 side bends.
17) Hold a towel in one hand with arms stretched out at side and bend till it touches floor 5 times.
18) Practice large golf swings for 20 strokes.

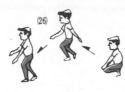

19) Swing arms front and back 20 times.
20) Push a wall for 5 seconds.
21) Open eyes wide and close tightly 5 times.
22) Stand on tiptoe and stretch back 10 times.
23) Carry a person of your own weight piggyback for 30 steps.
24) Run in figure eights for 1 minute.
25) Lift yourself from a chair with arms for 20 seconds.
26) Jump from a kneeling position with one leg.
27) Swing trunk in large circles in an erect kneeling position 10 times.
28) Do sit-ups with knees flexed 3 times.
29) Sprint 30 paces.
30) Flutter legs while lying on stomach 40 times for each leg.
31) Do 10 push-ups (women from knees).
32) Do one-handed push-ups with legs spread and one hand on back, touching forehead to hand 1 time for each hand.
33) In a push-up position with legs spread, cross and uncross legs in air.
34) Do a handstand with feet against a wall for 20 seconds.
35) Lying spread-eagled on back, tense and relax all muscles 10 times.
36) Stretch on floor in hurdling position 5 times.
37) Hold yourself in a frog position for 10 seconds.
38) Lie on back, lift legs over head, and touch toes to floor 10 times.
39) Do cycling exercises on back 30 times.
40) Lie on stomach and have partner stand on your arches 50 seconds.

"The instructor handed out a check sheet and told us to do as many of the forty tasks as possible in one hour, putting an X by the ones we couldn't do or didn't have time to do. We were told to do this in pairs, with one counting while the other did the tasks. It was difficult to judge how fast to go through the exercises. If we did them too fast, we would get tired quickly. If we did them too slowly, we wouldn't be able to finish.

"How many days, or rather months, has it been since I've worked my body so hard? I'm not totally exhausted, as I began to think I might be, but I feel kind of sluggish. The emphasis which the instructor put on physical fitness in his lecture makes real sense to me now. I intend to keep working on the exercise task sheet for at least the next six months.

"Tomorrow afternoon another session is scheduled, but this time we will get to use balls and other sports equipment. I'm looking forward to that. I'm just wondering how stiff I'm going to be in the morning."

Index

302